Pass the Texas Pharmacy Law Exam: A Study Guide and Review for the Texas MPJE

by Sarah Fichuk, Pharm.D., BCPS

Printed in the United States of America

First Printing, 2012
Second Printing, 2014

ISBN 978-0615655185

Straight A's Publishing

www.StraightAsPublishing.com

Table of Contents

Section One: Introduction...1
Test Overview 1
Laws and Rules Tested on the Texas MPJE®...........................1
When to Schedule Your Exams..2
Actually Taking the Test...3
Warning/Disclaimer 3
Make Sure You Know These!... 10
The "Golden Rule" for Pharmacy Law 11
Section Two: Federal Laws and Rules 15
Federal Food, Drug, and Cosmetic Act 15
Adultered 16
Misbranded.. 16
OTC Label Requirements 17
Other OTC Rules... 17
Recalls 17
Advertising... 18
Pregnancy Categories... 18
Plan B Rules 19
Section Three: Federal Controlled Substance Laws
.... 21
Schedule I Controlled Substances 21
Schedule II Controlled Substances...................................... 21
Schedule III Controlled Substances 22
Schedule IV Controlled Substances 22
Schedule V Controlled Substances...................................... 23
DEA Facts.. 23
DEA Registration 24
Prescriptions 24
Prescription Requirements... 25
DEA Registration Numbers... 25
Partial Refills of Schedule III, IV, and V.............................. 26
Refill Authorizations for Schedule III, IV, and V................... 26
Data Processing and Storage Requirements 26

DEA Form 222 27
Completing a DEA Form 222 27
Who May Sign a DEA Form 222? 27
Ordering Drugs Using DEA Form 222 28
Emergency Schedule II Prescriptions............................... 28
Transfer of Business 29
Disposing of Controlled Substances by a Reverse Distributor
.... 30
Disposing of Controlled Substances at a Pharmacy 30
Returning a Controlled Substance Prescription 30
Prescription Requirements.. 38
Changes to a Schedule II Prescription 38
Required Safety Features on Official Schedule II Prescription
Forms... 39
Partial Filling a Schedule II for a Long-Term Care Facility
(LTCF) or for a Terminally Ill Patient.. 42
Faxed Schedule II Prescriptions.. 42

**Section Five: Texas Controlled Substance Laws
Regarding Schedule III–V's** 45
Prescription Requirements.. 45
Records 47
Emergency Refills.. 47
Delivery of Controlled Substances..................................... 48
Designated Agents 48
Inspection 49
Discrepancies/Theft... 49
Automated Pharmacy System... 55
Telepharmacy System 56
Dispensing of Dangerous Drugs in Certain Rural Areas........ 57
Manufacturer Label Requirements...................................... 58

Section Eight: Texas Administrative Code................ 61
Grounds for Discipline for a Pharmacist License 61
Grounds for Discipline for a Pharmacy License 67
Grounds for Discipline for a Pharmacy Technician or a
Pharmacy Technician Trainee 68

Denial of a License 69
Reporting Professional Liability Claims 69
Section Nine: Pharmacists 71
Requirements to be a Licensed Pharmacist 71
Reciprocity Requirements 72
Emergency Temporary Pharmacist License 72
Pharmacist License Renewal 72
Continuing Education Requirements 73
Section Ten: Pharmacist-Interns 77
Hours 77
Student-Intern Requirements 77
Student-Intern Card 77
Pharmacist-Intern Identification 78
Intern Duties 78
Pharmacist-Interns May Not 79
Section Eleven: Preceptors 81
Requirements 81
Pharmacist Preceptor Requirements 81
Ratios 81
Section Twelve: Drug Therapy Management 83
Drug Therapy Management 83
Written Protocol 83
Performing Drug Therapy Management 84
Signing Prescriptions 85
Board Will Post on its Website 85
Pharmacist Training Requirements 85
Physician Requirements 85
Records 86
Written Protocol 86
Section Thirteen: Administration of
Immunizations or Vaccinations 87
Written Protocol 87
Pharmacist Certification Requirements 87
Supervision by Physician 88

Special Provisions 88
Notifications 88
Records 89

Section Fourteen: Pharmacy Technicians 91

Registration Requirements 91
Pharmacy Technician Trainee 91
Registration Requirements 92
Exemption from PTCB Examination 92
Registration Renewal 92
Continuing Education 92

Section Fifteen: Destruction of Dispensed Drugs 97

Drugs Dispensed to Patients in Healthcare Facilities 97
Destruction of Drugs Dispensed to Patients in Healthcare
Facilities by a Waste Disposal Service 98
Destruction by a Waste Disposal Service 99
Dangerous Drugs Returned to a Pharmacy 99
Disposal of Stock Prescription Drugs 100
Destruction of Stock Controlled Substances 100

Section Sixteen: Substitution of Drug Products . 103

Generic Substitution 103
Prohibiting Generic Substitution 103
Patient Notification 104
Records 104
Determining Generic Equivalency 105

Section Seventeen: Laws Regarding Pharmacies

.... 107
Display Requirements 107
Required Notifications to the Board 107
Closing a Pharmacy 108
Recalls 108
Return of Prescription Drugs 109
Pick up of Prescriptions 109
Samples 109
Inventory Requirements 110
Professional Responsibility of Pharmacists 111

Section Eighteen: Class A Pharmacy Rules........... 113
Personnel.. 113
Pharmacist Duties.. 113
Pharmacy Technician/Trainee Duties 114
Technician Ratios 114
Identification of Pharmacy Personnel.................... 115
Operational Standards 115
Security.. 116
Temporary Absence of Pharmacist – On-Site 117
Temporary Absence of a Pharmacist – Off-Site..... 118
Patient Counseling.. 118
Counseling Must be Provided 119
Drug Regimen Review.. 120
Substitution of Dosage Form.................................... 121
Prescription Containers 121
Labeling Requirements on a Prescription to be Dispensed
.... 121
Returning Undelivered Medication to Stock 122
Equipment and Supplies 123
Drugs.. 124
Customized Patient Medication Packages – Med-Pak 124
Automated Compounding or Counting Devices and Systems
.... 125
Automated Storage and Distribution Device......... 125
Maintenance of Records 126
Prescriptions 127
Prescription Drug Orders Written by Out of State
Practitioners.. 127
Prescriptions Written by Practitioners in Mexico or Canada
.... 128
Prescriptions Carried Out or Signed by an Advanced Practice
Nurse, Physician Assistant, or Pharmacist............ 128
Verbal Prescriptions 129
Electronic Prescriptions for Dangerous Drugs..... 129
Prescription Records 130

Prescription Requirements 130
Pharmacist Documentation on Prescriptions 131
Refills 132
Auto-Refill Program 134
Dispensing 90-Day Supply 134
Transfers 135
Data Processing Systems 138
Distribution of Controlled Substances 139
Records 139

Section Nineteen: Class B – Nuclear Pharmacy Rules 141

Owner 141
Pharmacist-In-Charge 141
Qualifications of Nuclear Pharmacists 142
Technician Ratios 142
Library 142

Section Twenty: Class C Institutional Pharmacy Rules 145

Pharmacist Requirements 145
Pharmacist-In-Charge (PIC) 145
Pharmacist Duties 145
Technician Duties in a Facility with ≥101 Beds 146
Technician Duties in a Facility with ≤100 beds 147
Tech-Check-Tech 148
Rural Hospitals 149
Identification of Pharmacy Personnel 150
Library 150
Removing Drugs When Pharmacy Closed 151
Floor Stock 151
Formulary 152
Prepackaging Drugs to be Kept at Facility 152
Sterile Preparations Prepared Outside the Pharmacy 152
Medication Orders 153
Discharge Prescriptions 153
Drug Regimen Review 154

Dispensing Take Home Medications from the ER.................. 154
Dispensing Drugs to Radiology Outpatients........................... 155
Automated Devices and Systems... 156
Automated Medication Supply Systems Used for Storage and
Recordkeeping of Medications Located Outside of the
Pharmacy Department (Pyxis)... 157
Maintenance of Records.. 158
Outpatient Records.. 159
Original Medication Orders 160
Patient Medication Records (PMR) 160
Loss of Data.. 160
Distribution of Controlled Substances to Another Registrant
.... 161
Other Records to be Maintained by a Pharmacy 162
Permission to Maintain Central Records 163

**Section Twenty-One: Class C Pharmacies Located
in a Freestanding Ambulatory Surgical Center
(ASC) Rules**.. 167
Personnel.. 167
Operational Standards 167
Library 167

**Section Twenty-Seven: Services Provided by
Pharmacies**.. 251
Remote Pharmacy Services... 251
General Requirements 251
Operational Standards 252
Environment/Security of Automated Pharmacy System... 253
Prescription Dispensing and Delivery 253
Stocking an Automated Pharmacy System........................... 253
Quality Assurance Program 254
Records.. 254
Inventory 255
Emergency Medication Kits.. 255
Definitions.. 255

General Requirements 256
Operational Standards 257
Notification Requirements 257
Environment/Security 258
Prescription Drugs and Delivery 258
Drugs 258
Stocking Emergency Medication Kits 259
Inventory 260
Telepharmacy 260
Definitions 260
General Requirements 261
Operational Standards 262
Notification Requirements 263
Environment/Security 263
Prescription Dispensing and Delivery 264
Quality Assurance Program 266
Inventory 266
**Central Prescription Drug or Medication Order
Processing** 267
Definition 267
Operational Standards 267
Notifications to Patients 268
Records 269
Centralized Prescription Dispensing 269
Definition 269
Operational Standards 270
Notifications to Patients 270
Prescription Labeling 271
Records 272

**Section Twenty-Nine: Compounding Sterile
Preparations** 285
Pharmacy Technicians and Pharmacy Technician Trainees
Training Prior to September 1, 2015 290

Pharmacy Technicians and Pharmacy Technician Trainees Training Effective September 1, 2015............................ 291

Operational Standards 299

Other Rules 299

Microbial Contamination Risk Levels........................... 300

    Low-risk level compounded sterile preparations............ 300

    Low-Risk Level compounded sterile preparations with 12-hour or fewer beyond-use date................................... 301

    Medium-risk level compounded sterile preparations 301

    High-risk level compounded sterile preparations........... 303

    Immediate Use Compounded Sterile Preparations......... 304

Library 306

Environment... 306

Cytotoxic Drugs... 307

Cleaning and Disinfecting the Sterile Compounding Areas 307

Labeling.. 310

Personnel Cleansing and Garbing 310

Section Thirty: Pseudoephederine Laws................. 325

Definitions.. 335

Law Review Questions 379

Section One: Introduction

Test Overview

- Online registration at www.nabp.net
- Computer-based test
- Adaptive technology selects the next question based on the answers to your previous questions
- No distinction between federal and Texas law (answer according to the strictest rule)
- 2 hours for 90 questions
- 75 scored questions
- 15 pretest questions
- Scored questions are not identified
- Minimum passing score is 75 in a range of 0–100
- Scaled score (compares your score to the minimum acceptable score)
- Cannot change an answer once it has been confirmed
- Cannot go back and review questions
- All questions must be answered in order
- Cannot skip questions
- Scores are available online at www.nabp.net within 7 business days (usually in 2-3 business days)

Laws and Rules Tested on the Texas MPJE®

- Texas Pharmacy Act
- Texas Dangerous Drug Act
- Texas Pharmacy Rules (Texas Administrative Code)
- Federal Food, Drug and Cosmetic Act
- Texas Food, Drug and Cosmetic Act
- Federal Controlled Substance Act
- Poison Prevention Packaging Act

How to Study

I recommend that you make sure you read the sections **Make Sure You Know These!** and **Test Objectives** prior to reading through the chapters so you know what information to pay special attention to while studying. Everything is important, but there are certain things you must know.

I suggest you read through the chapters at least **3** times, then go back to the **Make Sure You Know These!** list and make sure you can answer each one as if it were a question. Only go through the practice questions after you have read through the chapters a few times. The practice questions will help identify areas that you may need to review.

Particularly focus on all the information in the controlled substances sections. Read those sections again just prior to taking the test. It would be better to be over-prepared rather than underprepared. This is one of the most important tests of your career.

When to Schedule Your Exams

I recommend focusing on only one exam at time, either the NAPLEX® or the MPJE®. You will probably need a minimum of a week to study for the MPJE®, if not two weeks. So keep that in mind when scheduling your exams.

Actually Taking the Test

There will be answers like "1 and 2," "2 only," and "1, 2 and 3."

Read each question carefully. Do not read too much into the question or try to overanalyze—think in straightforward terms and go with your first choice when reading the answers.

Do not rush through each question. You have plenty of time to take the test—over a minute for each question—and some will be easy and straightforward, so don't panic about time. Some questions, you have to guess at, so don't get discouraged.

Warning/Disclaimer

This book is not intended to be comprehensive review of all pharmacy law. Many of the rules and laws applicable to the practice of pharmacy were **NOT** included because the author felt they were unlikely to be on the Texas MPJE®. This book is a study guide to help pharmacists and pharmacy students pass the Texas MPJE®. It is intended to be a supplement to the law class taken in pharmacy school.

If the reader has concerns over a statement made in this book or has further questions, the reader should read the actual law referenced.

A word of caution: Even if you have worked retail as a technician for years, you still need to study to pass this test. The pharmacy you worked at may not have been following the law as written.

Test Objectives

Texas Pharmacy Act
- Purpose of the Board
- Definitions
- Board membership/makeup
- Board responsibilities
- Board inspections
- Unlawful practice of pharmacy
- Pharmacist-intern registration
- Licensure examination
- Licensing by exam and reciprocity
- Display requirements for pharmacist licensure
- Pharmacist license renewal
- Continuing education requirements
- Pharmacist license inactivity
- Discipline of a pharmacist's or pharmacy's license
- Discipline in a Class E pharmacy
- Temporary suspension of a pharmacist or pharmacy's license
- License and renewal of pharmacy license
- Time limits for notification to Board
- Administration and provision of dangerous drugs
- Unlawful use of the words "pharmacy" and "pharmacist"
- Drug substitution
- Emergency refills
- Release of confidential records
- Operation of remote pharmacy services

Texas Pharmacy Rules of Procedure
- Grounds for disciplining a pharmacist's license
- Goals of internship
- Reissue of a license

4

- Removal of restrictions on a license
- Extended internship program
- Duties of a pharmacist-intern
- Preceptor requirements
- Examination and reciprocity requirements
- Renewal of an expired license
- Procedure for change of name, location, ownership, or managing officers of a pharmacy
- Closure of a pharmacy
- Return of dispensed prescription drugs
- Locations of prescription pick-up
- Balance registration
- Discussion of the terms "failure to engage in the business described in the application for a license" and "ceased to engage in the business described in the application for a license"
- Description of the responsibilities of the pharmacist-in-charge of a pharmacy that experiences a fire or other disaster;
- Theft or loss of a controlled substance or dangerous drug
- Requirements for inventory
- Personnel, operation standards, and record keeping for
  - Class A (Community) Pharmacy
  - Class B (Nuclear) Pharmacy
  - Class C (Institutional) Pharmacy
  - Class C (Institutional) Pharmacy Located in a Freestanding Ambulatory Surgical Center
  - Class D (Clinic) Pharmacy
  - Class E (Non-Resident) Pharmacy
- Pharmacy technicians and trainees: ratios, duties, and training in each class of pharmacy
- Pharmacist-in-charge responsibilities in each class

- Patient counseling and providing drug information in Class A
- Patient medication record requirements in Class A and C
- Drug regimen review in Class A and C
- Personnel identification in Class A and C
- Security requirements
- Temporary absence (on- and off-site) of a pharmacist in Class A
- Prescription filling system
- Written, verbal, and fax prescription requirements
- Prescription label requirements
- Automation of pharmacy procedure
- Refill requirements for controlled substances and dangerous drugs
- Documenting refill authorization
- Telephone and electronic prescription transfer
- Schedule II official prescription requirements and exceptions
- Prescription requirements and restrictions on practitioners not licensed in Texas
- Drug therapy management and vaccine administration
- Prescriptions by advanced practice nurses and physician assistants
- Class A pharmacy requirements that compounds sterile/non-sterile items
- Pharmacy requirements if doing central prescription processing
- Inpatient records in a Class C pharmacy
- Supplying drugs from an emergency room
- Dispensing prescriptions to outpatients of a hospital
- Record requirements for Schedule II and floor stock in Class C
- Class D drug/device formulary and how to expand

- Pharmacist supervision in Class D
- Class E pharmacies mailing to Texas residents
- Automated pharmacy system
- Telepharmacy system
- Emergency medication kits
- Requirements for continuing education
- Placing license on inactive status
- Destruction of dispensed drugs
- Destruction of stock drugs
- Generic substitution
- Board Certification
- Use of automation in a pharmacy

Federal and State Controlled Substance Acts and Regulations

- Definitions of controlled substances
- Who registers with DEA and DPS and how
- Storage requirements for controlled substances
- What records must be maintained
- Central record keeping requirements and restrictions
- Obtaining, executing, and storing DEA order forms
- Returning controlled substances to supplier
- Disposing expired or contaminated controlled substances
- Prescription requirements for Schedule II–V
- Refill requirements for Schedule II–V
- Emergency refill requirements for Schedule III–V
- Partial dispensing of Schedule II and Schedule III–V
- Emergency oral order of Schedule II
- Federal "transfer warning" statement
- OTC sale of Schedule V products
- Schedule II prescription requirements and exceptions
- Criteria to place a drug in the five schedules

- Recognizing commonly used controlled substances and their schedules
- Reporting theft/loss to DEA and DPS
- Employee screening
- Procedures for closing a business
- Legal use of methadone
- Methadone to treat addiction
- Using Subutex® or Suboxone®
- Physicians' designated agents
- Schedule II prescription written by a practitioner not licensed in Texas
- Faxed Schedule II prescriptions

Federal and State Food, Drug, and Cosmetic Acts
- Definitions
- Adultered
- Misbranded
- Registration requirements for manufacturers and distributors
- Illegal pharmacist acts under the Durham-Humphrey Amendments
- Requirements for manufacturers' labels
- How long to keep prescriptions
- Recall classification system
- Good Manufacturing Practice

Texas Dangerous Drug Act
- Prescription labeling requirements
- Refilling a prescription
- Who can possess dangerous drugs
- Records to be maintained
- Primary enforcing agency

- Forgery
- Physicians' designated agents

Miscellaneous
- Exceptions to child-resistant packaging
- Mailing controlled substances
- Prescribing restrictions by therapeutic optometrists

Make Sure You Know These!

- Know time frames for everything
  - When to report to the DEA, DPS, and board
  - How long to keep records
  - How long to keep CE records
- Emergency kits
- Everything on controlled substances
- DEA form numbers
- Know the common definitions, like *adultered* and *misbranded*
- Automated pharmacy systems
- Telepharmacy/remote pharmacy services
- Childproof containers
- Prescribing methadone
- Pharmacy technician ratios and training requirements
- Buying Plan B
- Prescription label requirements
- Changes to a Schedule II prescription
- Counseling requirements
- Drugs that can be prescribed by a therapeutic optometrist
- Pharmacist-intern and pharmacy technician duties
- Reporting professional liability claims
- Preceptor requirements
- Pharmacist administration of vaccines
- Physician dispensing
- Sterile compounding – the different risk levels and expiration dates

The "Golden Rule" for Pharmacy Law

You are required to follow the strictest standard when comparing federal and state law. For example federal law allows 3 different filing systems for prescriptions but Texas only allows 1. Therefore the correct standard to follow is the Texas law.

Also keep all records for a minimum of 2 years and keep CE records for 3 years

Acronyms

ACPE – Accreditation Council for Pharmacy Education
ACLS – Advanced Cardiac Life Support
BCLS – Basic Cardiac Life Support
CE – continuing education
DEA – Drug Enforcement Administration
DPS – Department of Public Safety
FDA – Food and Drug Administration
FPGEC – Foreign Pharmacy Graduate Equivalency Commission
FPGEE – Foreign Pharmacy Graduate Equivalency Examination
GED – General Education Development
HEPA – High efficiency particulate air
HIPAA – Health Insurance Portability and Accountability Act
IPA – Isopropyl alcohol
ISO – International Organization of Standardization
MPJE – Multistate Pharmacy Jurisprudence Examination
MSA – Metropolitan statistical area
NABP – National Association of Boards of Pharmacy
NAPLEX – North American Pharmacy Licensing Examination
NDC – national drug code
OTC – Over the counter
PALS – Pediatric Advanced Life Support
PIC – pharmacist-in-charge
PMR – Patient medication record
PTCB – Pharmacy Technician Certification Board
SOP – Standard operating procedure
SWFI – Sterile water for injection
TPN – total potential nutrition
TSBP – Texas State Board of Pharmacy
USP/NF – United States Pharmacopeia/National Formulary

Section Two: Federal Laws and Rules

Federal Food, Drug, and Cosmetic Act

Purpose: protect the public health by requiring safe, effective, and properly labeled drugs and devices

History

- **1906 Pure Food and Drug Act**
  - Purity standards only; no efficacy requirements
- **1938 Federal Food, Drug, and Cosmetic Act**
  - Safety standards only; no efficacy requirements
- **1951 Durham-Humphrey Amendments**
  - Created OTC and prescription drug categories
- **1962 Kefauver-Harris Amendment**
  - Efficacy requirements
- **1976 Medical Device Amendment**
  - Added regulatory authority over devices
- **1983 Orphan Drug Act**
  - Incentives to create drugs for rare diseases (longer patent life)
- **1984 Drug Price Competition and Patent Restoration Act**
  - Patent holders received 5 years of patent life because of the FDA's process to review drug applications
- **1988 Prescription Drug Marketing Act of 1987**
  - State licensing of wholesale distributors
  - Banned reimportation of prescription drugs
  - Banned sale, trade, or purchase of drug samples
- **1997 FDA Modernization Act**
  - Requires "Rx only" on the prescription legend
- **1999 Over-the-Counter Labeling Requirements**
  - Standardized OTC labeling

Adultered

Refers to the actual makeup or composition of the drug
- Containing any filthy substance
- May have been contaminated in preparation/storage/packaging
- Good manufacturing practices not followed
- Container may contaminate the drug
- Unsafe color additive
- Strength differs from what listed on the label (A 5% difference is okay)
- Misfilled: drug has been substituted

Misbranded

Refers to the drug labeling
- Labeling is false or misleading
- Manufacturer's labeling requirements:
  - Name and address of manufacturer
  - Quantity
  - Generic and brand name of the drug (if applicable)
  - Strength of the drug
  - Information for use
  - Warnings against use
  - Expiration date
- Pharmacist filling a prescription without authorization from prescriber
- Counterfeit drug
- Packaging violates Poison Prevention Packaging Act
- Packaging not containing all the words or statements as required by law

OTC Label Requirements

- Must contain adequate *directions* for use—in comparison, prescription drug labeling must contain adequate *information* for use
- Display panel with name of product
- Name and address of manufacturer/packer/distributor
- Quantity in container
- Cautions and warnings
- Adequate directions for safe and effective use (must be written for a layperson)
- "Drug Facts" must contain
    - Active ingredients
    - Purpose
    - Uses – indications
    - Warnings
    - Directions
    - Other information
    - Inactive ingredients
    - Questions? (optional) followed by telephone number

Other OTC Rules

- Prescribed an OTC but dose is higher than OTC limits: must be written and filled as a prescription
- If an OTC is written as a prescription, then it needs to be filled as a prescription, but a pharmacist can sell an OTC if he or she feels it to be in the best interest of the patient

Recalls

- FDA has no authority to recall drugs, only devices
- **Class I recall** – reasonable probability exposure will cause serious adverse health effects or death

- **Class II recall** – may cause temporary or medically reversible adverse health effects
- **Class III recall** – not likely to cause adverse health effects

Advertising
- Prescription drug advertising – regulated by FDA
- OTC advertising – regulated by Federal Trade Commission
- Pharmacists may advertise
  - Provide pricing information—must include brand/generic name, strength, dosage form, and price charged for a specific quantity
  - Availability of professional services
  - Price stated must include all charges to consumer; mailing and delivery fees may be stated separately

Pregnancy Categories

Category A
Adequate and well-controlled studies have failed to demonstrate a risk to the fetus in the first trimester of pregnancy (and there is no evidence of risk in later trimesters).

Category B
Animal reproduction studies have failed to demonstrate a risk to the fetus, and there are no adequate and well-controlled studies in pregnant women.

Category C
Animal reproduction studies have shown an adverse effect on the fetus, and there are no adequate and well-controlled

studies in humans, but potential benefits may warrant use of the drug in pregnant women despite potential risks.

Category D
There is positive evidence of human fetal risk based on adverse reaction data from investigational or marketing experience or studies in humans, but potential benefits may warrant use of the drug in pregnant women despite potential risks.

Category X
Studies in animals or humans have demonstrated fetal abnormalities and/or there is positive evidence of human fetal risk based on adverse reaction data from investigational or marketing experience, and the risks involved in use of the drug in pregnant women clearly outweigh potential benefits.

Plan B Rules

- Plan B, Plan B One-Step, and their generic versions are allowed to be sold over-the-counter to consumers 17 years and older and available by prescription only for women 16 years and younger
- Only sold in pharmacies/stores staffed by a licensed pharmacist
- Will be kept behind the pharmacy counter because the packaging has both over-the-counter and prescription labeling
- Proof of age via personal identification will be required at time of purchase
- Men may purchase Plan B—the wording is "to consumers 17 years and older"

Section Three: Federal Controlled Substance Laws

Schedule I Controlled Substances

- High potential for abuse
- No currently accepted medical use
- Lack of accepted safety for use under medical supervision
- Examples:
  - Heroin
  - Lysergic acid diethylamide (LSD)
  - Marijuana (cannabis)
  - Peyote
  - 3,4-methylenedioxymethamphetamine ("ecstasy")
- ** Use of peyote by the Native American Church is allowed, but manufacturers and distributors of peyote must be registered

Schedule II Controlled Substances

- High potential for abuse which may lead to severe psychological or physical dependence
- Examples:
  - Narcotics
    - Hydromorphone (Dilaudid®)
    - Methadone (Dolophine®)
    - Meperidine (Demerol®)
    - Oxycodone (OxyContin®)
    - Fentanyl (Sublimaze® or Duragesic®)
  - Stimulants

- Amphetamine (Dexedrine®, Adderall®)
- Methamphetamine (Desoxyn®)
- Methylphenidate (Ritalin®)
  - Others
    - Cocaine
    - Amobarbital
    - Glutethimide
    - Pentobarbital

Schedule III Controlled Substances

- Potential for abuse less than substances in schedules I or II and abuse may lead to moderate or low physical dependence or high psychological dependence
- Examples:
  - Narcotics
    - Combination products containing less than 15 milligrams of hydrocodone per dosage unit (Vicodin®)
    - Products containing not more than 90 milligrams of codeine per dosage unit (Tylenol with codeine®)
  - Products to treat opioid addiction
    - Buprenorphine (Suboxone® and Subutex®)
  - Others
    - Benzphetamine (Didrex®)
    - Phendimetrazine
    - Ketamine
    - Anabolic steroids

Schedule IV Controlled Substances

- Low potential for abuse relative to substances in Schedule III

- Effective 1/11/12: carisoprodol will be Schedule IV
- Examples:
    - Alprazolam (Xanax®)
    - Clonazepam (Klonopin®)
    - Clorazepate (Tranxene®)
    - Diazepam (Valium®)
    - Lorazepam (Ativan®)
    - Midazolam (Versed®)
    - Temazepam (Restoril®)
    - Triazolam (Halcion®)

Schedule V Controlled Substances

- Low potential for abuse relative to substances listed in schedule IV
- Contain limited quantities of certain narcotics
- Generally used for antitussive, antidiarrheal, and analgesic purposes
- Examples
    - Cough preparations containing not more than 200 milligrams of codeine per 100 milliliters or per 100 grams (Robitussin AC® and Phenergan with Codeine®)

DEA Facts

- The U.S. Drug Enforcement Administration (DEA) is a component of the U.S. Department of Justice
- "responsible for enforcing the controlled substances laws and regulations of the United States"

DEA Registration

- All DEA registrants: register every 3 years with DEA form 224 (for pharmacies)
- DEA sends out renewal form 60 days prior to expiration date
- Must notify DEA in writing if have not received renewal form 45 days prior to expiration date

Prescriptions

- Must be for legitimate medical purposes
- Practitioner must be acting in the usual course of their professional practice
- Pharmacists also have a corresponding responsibility with the practitioner for the proper prescribing and dispensing
- Writing a prescription "for office use" is not allowed; practitioner must order directly from a supplier or distributor
- Narcotic prescriptions may not be written for "detoxification treatment" or "maintenance treatment"
- Physicians should not write prescriptions for themselves or family members (but no law against it)
- Practitioners do not need to register with the DEA if they work at a hospital/institution (can use the hospital's DEA number and then the code assigned to them)
- Schedule III–V are allowed 5 refills in the 6 months from the date written

Prescription Requirements

- A prescription must be written in ink or indelible pencil or typewritten and must be manually signed by the practitioner
- A prescription for a controlled substance must include the following information:
  - Date of issue
  - Patient's name and address
  - Practitioner's name, address, and DEA registration number
  - Drug name
  - Drug strength
  - Dosage form
  - Quantity prescribed
  - Directions for use
  - Number of refills (if any) authorized; and
  - Manual signature of prescriber

DEA Registration Numbers

There is an easy formula to determine if a DEA number is valid
- Add the 1st, 3rd, and 5th digits of the DEA number
- Add the 2nd, 4th and 6th digits and multiply by 2
- Add the results of those two calculations
- The last digit from the sum of the first two steps should be the same as the 7th digit in the DEA number
- Example: BF1234563
  - $1 + 3 + 5 = 9$
  - $2 + 4 + 6 = 12 \times 2 = 24$
  - $9 + 24 = 33$
  - So the 7th digit should be "3"
  - Therefore this DEA number is valid

Partial Refills of Schedule III, IV, and V

Partial refills are allowed, provided that each partial filling is dispensed and recorded in the same manner as a refilling (e.g., date refilled, amount dispensed, initials of dispensing pharmacist), the total quantity dispensed in all partial fillings does not exceed the total quantity prescribed, and no dispensing occurs after 6 months past the date of issue.

Refill Authorizations for Schedule III, IV, and V

- Prescriber allowed to orally authorize additional refills
- Not allowed to exceed 5 refills in a 6-month time period from the date the prescription was originally written
- Quantity of each additional refill must be the same as or less than the initial quantity authorized
- New and separate prescription required for any additional quantities above and beyond the "5 refills in 6 months" limit

Data Processing and Storage Requirements

- Pharmacists are allowed to store refill information in a computer
- System must produce a daily hard copy readout of all processed controlled substance refills
- Each individual pharmacist must verify the information is correct and date and sign the hard copy readout
- A logbook may be used instead of the daily hard copy readout, where each pharmacist must sign a statement every day that says the information entered into the computer that day was correct

DEA Form 222

- Required for the sale or transfer of Schedule I or II controlled substances
- Pharmacies may transfer controlled substances to other pharmacies as long as the total amount is up to 5% of the total amount of controlled substances dispensed in a year without having to register as a wholesaler
- Carbon triplicate: Copy 1, Copy 2, and Copy 3
- Each form is numbered serially
- Preprinted with name, address, and registration number of the registrant; the authorized activity; and the schedules of the registrant
  - Cannot be changed
  - In case of changed information, must have new forms made

Completing a DEA Form 222

- Must be completed in ink, indelible pencil, or typewritten
- Only one item per numbered line on the form
  - "One item" means one drug, strength, and package size
- The number of lines completed must be filled in at the bottom of the form
- Name and address of the supplier must be filled in

Who May Sign a DEA Form 222?

- Individual who signed the DEA registration
- Individual who is authorized through the execution of a power of attorney by an individual who signed the DEA registration

Ordering Drugs Using DEA Form 222

- Purchaser fills out the form and submits Copy 1 and 2 to the supplier and keeps Copy 3 for their records
- Supplier fills the order and records on Copy 1 and 2 the number of commercial or bulk containers supplied on each item and the date shipped to purchaser
- Order may be filled in part, with the balance shipped within 60 days of the date on the form
- After 60 days, the order form is no longer valid
- May only be shipped to the address on the form
- Supplier keeps Copy 1 and forwards Copy 2 to the DEA
- When the purchaser receives the shipment, they must note how many containers received on each item and the date received on Copy 3
- Order form may not be filled if it
  - Is not complete, legible, or properly prepared, executed, or endorsed
  - Shows any adulteration, erasure, or change of any description

Emergency Schedule II Prescriptions

- DEA regulations limit an emergency oral prescription to the quantity necessary to treat the patient during the emergency period
- Oral emergency prescriptions must immediately be reduced to writing by the pharmacist and must contain all the information ordinarily required in a prescription, except for the signature of the prescribing individual practitioner
- If the prescribing individual practitioner is not known to the pharmacist, the pharmacist must make a reasonable effort to determine that the oral authorization came from a registered individual

practitioner, which may include a call back to the prescribing individual practitioner and/or other good faith efforts to ensure the practitioner's identity
- An emergency situation is defined as all of the following:
  - Immediate administration of the controlled substance is necessary for proper treatment
  - No appropriate alternative treatments are available including non–Schedule II controlled substances
  - Not reasonably possible for the physician to provide a written prescription prior to dispensing

Transfer of Business

- Notify DEA 14 days prior to transfer
- Day of transfer: complete inventory, which serves as both the closing and opening inventories
- Transferring schedule II – use official DEA 222 order form
- Transferring schedule III–V – separate document with
  - Name of drug
  - Dosage form
  - Strength
  - Quantity
  - Date transferred
  - Names, addresses, and DEA numbers of the pharmacies

Disposing of Controlled Substances by a Reverse Distributor

- May send to a reverse distributor registered with the DEA
    - Schedule II – DEA 222
    - Schedule III–V – written record of name, form, strength, quantity
- Reverse distributor will submit to the DEA form 41 when the controlled substances have been destroyed
- Disposal by those **not** registered with the DEA (ex. long-term care facilities)

Disposing of Controlled Substances at a Pharmacy

- Once a year, retail pharmacies may request DEA permission to dispose of controlled substances that are unwanted, expired, etc.
- Pharmacy completes DEA Form 41 that lists all drugs to be destroyed
- Pharmacy sends letter to DEA with the form at least 14 days in advance, asking for permission
    - Letter contains the proposed date of destruction, method of destruction, and identity of the two witnesses (licensed physician, pharmacist, mid-level practitioner, nurse, or state or local law enforcement officer)

Returning a Controlled Substance Prescription

- An individual may not return unused controlled substance prescription medication to the pharmacy
- There are no provisions in federal laws and regulations to acquire controlled substances from a non-registrant (e.g., individual patient)

- An individual may dispose of their own controlled substance medication without approval from DEA

Theft or Significant Loss
- Notify DEA within one business day of the discovery
- Notify local law enforcement and state regulatory agencies
- Complete DEA form 106

Inventory Requirements
- Actual count of Schedule II
- Estimate count of Schedule III, IV, and V if bottle is <1,000 count
- Actual count of Schedule III, IV, and V if bottle >1,000 count
- Keep records for 2 years
- Records and inventories of Schedule I and II must be kept separately from all other records
- Records and inventories of Schedule III, IV, and V must be kept separately from all other records or readily retrievable
- Inventory of all controlled substances must be done every 2 years

Authorized Agent of the Prescriber
- An authorized agent of the prescriber may
  - Prepare a controlled substance prescription for the signature of the prescriber
  - Orally communicated a prescriber's Schedule III–V prescription to a pharmacist
  - Transmit by fax a prescriber's written Schedule II prescription to a pharmacist
- An authorized agent **cannot** orally communicate an emergency Schedule II prescription to a pharmacist

- To be an agent of the prescriber, a detailed written document must be created and specifies the authority being granted
- DEA also recommends providing a copy to pharmacies likely to receive prescriptions from the prescriber's agent
- Pharmacists still retain responsibility to make sure the controlled substance prescription conforms to the appropriate laws and regulations and is for a legitimate medical purpose

Electronic Prescribing of Controlled Substances
- Practitioners may write electronic controlled substance prescriptions
- Pharmacies may receive, dispense, and archive these electronic prescriptions
- Pharmacies must use specific software approved by the DEA, which must be certified by a third party audit

Central Filling of Controlled Substances
- Central fill pharmacies are permitted to fill the initial and refills of Schedule II, III, IV, and V prescriptions
- May be transmitted electronically or via fax from the community pharmacy
- Community pharmacy writes "CENTRAL FILL" on the face of the original prescription and includes name, address and DEA number of the central fill pharmacy
- Central fill pharmacies must place a label to the packaging showing the local pharmacy name and address as well as a unique identifier to show it was filled at the central fill pharmacy

Prescribing Methadone for Pain

- Federal law and regulations do not restrict the prescribing, dispensing, or administering of any schedule II, III, IV, or V narcotic medication, including methadone, for the treatment of pain, if such treatment is deemed medically necessary by a registered practitioner acting in the usual course of professional practice.
- Use of methadone for the maintenance or detoxification of opioid-addicted individuals, in which case the practitioner is required to be registered with the DEA as a Narcotic Treatment Program (NTP)

Detoxification or Maintenance Treatment

- A practitioner may administer or dispense directly (but not prescribe) a narcotic drug listed in any schedule to a narcotic-dependent person for the purpose of maintenance or detoxification treatment if the practitioner meets both of the following conditions:
  - is separately registered with DEA as a narcotic treatment program
  - complies with DEA regulations regarding treatment qualifications, security, records, and unsupervised use of the drugs
- A physician who is not specifically registered to conduct a narcotic treatment program may administer (but not prescribe) narcotic drugs to a person for the purpose of relieving acute withdrawal symptoms when necessary while arrangements are being made for referral for treatment.
  - No more than 1 day's medication may be administered to the person or for the person's use at one time.

- Such emergency treatment may be carried out for no more than 3 days and may not be renewed or extended.
- Physicians may administer or dispense narcotic drugs in a hospital to maintain or detoxify a person as an incidental adjunct to a medical or surgical treatment of conditions other than addiction or those with intractable pain

Transferring Controlled Substance Prescriptions

- Allowed one time only
  - If pharmacies electronically share a real-time, online database, pharmacies may transfer up to the maximum refills permitted
- Must be communicated directly between two licensed pharmacists
- Transferring pharmacist
  - Voids the prescription
  - Records the name, address, and DEA number of the pharmacy to which it was transferred
  - Records the name of the pharmacist receiving the prescription
  - Records the date of the transfer and name of the pharmacist performing the transfer
- Receiving pharmacist writes
  - "Transfer" on the face of the prescription
  - Date of issuance of original prescription
  - Original number of refills authorized
  - Date of original dispensing
  - Number of valid refills remaining and date(s) and locations of previous refill(s)
  - Pharmacy's name, address, DEA number, and prescription number from which the prescription was transferred

- Name of pharmacist who transferred the prescription
- Pharmacy's name, address, DEA number, and prescription number from which the prescription was originally filled

Section Four: Texas Controlled Substance Laws Regarding Schedule II's

Registration
- Must notify DPS before day **7** after any change in
  - business name
  - address
  - physician delegating prescriptive authority
  - telephone number
  - other information required on the application, registration, or permit
- Must register in order to manufacture, distribute, prescribe, possess, analyze, dispense, or conduct research with a controlled substance
- Must apply after registering with the DEA
- Must display at the place of business
- Must register every year

Schedule II Prescriptions
- Must use an official Texas prescription form
- No refills allowed
- Only one prescription per official prescription form
- Prescription must be filled no later than 21 days after the date of issuance
- Multiple prescriptions: must ensure each prescription is not filled prior to the earliest date intended by the practitioner or 21 days after earliest date the prescription may be filled
- Is void if presented for filling 21 days after issuance or 21 days after any earliest fill date
- May issue multiple prescriptions

- o Up to a 90-day supply
- o Must be for a legitimate medical purpose
- o Must include the earliest date on which a pharmacy may fill
- o Must not cause risk of diversion or abuse

Prescription Requirements
- Practitioner must include
  - o Date written
  - o Controlled substance prescribed
  - o Quantity (written as both a number and word)
  - o Intended use or diagnosis
  - o Instructions for use
  - o Practitioner's name, address, DPS number, DEA number
  - o Patient's name, address, date of birth (or age)
  - o Earliest date on which it can be filled (if to be filled at a later date)
  - o Signature
- Pharmacist must include
  - o Date filled
  - o Signature
- Not more than one prescription per official prescription form

Changes to a Schedule II Prescription
As of 10/31/08 the TSBP and DPS have agreed the following may **not** be changed on a Schedule II prescription:
- Name of the patient
- Name of the drug
- Name of the prescribing physician
- Date of the prescription

Anything else may be changed on the prescription (such as strength of drug, quantity, directions for use) as long as the pharmacist

- Obtains verbal permission from the prescribing physician
- Documents on the prescription
    - Change that was authorized
    - Name or initials of individual giving authorization
    - Initial of the pharmacist

Required Safety Features on Official Schedule II Prescription Forms

All four safety features are required on each prescription

1. Control Number – in uppermost corner, unique to each prescription form
2. Pantograph – resulting in the word "VOID" in several places on the face of prescription when copied
3. Thermochromic Ink – on the back of the prescription form to show the word "SAFE" or to hide the check mark when rubbed
4. DPS Seal –a watermark on the face of the prescription

Dispensing an Emergency Quantity of a Schedule II upon Discharge

May dispense a Schedule II to a patient that is admitted to the hospital** and will require an emergency quantity upon release

- Properly labeled container
- Max 7-day supply or the minimum amount needed for proper treatment until patient can go to a pharmacy—whichever is less

- **Hospital* – a general hospital, special hospital, licensed ambulatory surgical center, surgical suite in a dental school, or veterinary medical school
  - May refer to a hospital clinic or emergency room, if the clinic or emergency room is under the control, direction, and administration as an integral part of a general or special hospital

Official Schedule II Prescription Form Not Required

- Someone admitted to a hospital
- A long-term care facility (LCTF) when
  - Administered from the facility's medical emergency kit
  - Administered by an authorized practitioner or an agent acting under the practitioner's order
  - Facility maintains proper records as required for an emergency medical kit in a LCTF
- An animal admitted to an animal hospital
- Member of a life flight helicopter medical team or an emergency medical ambulance crew or a paramedic-emergency medical technician and considered an extension of an emergency room of a general or special hospital
- Inmate in a correctional facility
- Therapeutic optometrist administering a topical ocular pharmaceutical agent

Submitting Prescription Information to DPS

Must submit information from Schedule II prescriptions to the DPS

- Prescribing practitioner's DPS registration number
- Official prescription control number

- Patient's (or animal owner's) name, age (or date of birth), and address (including city, state, and ZIP code)
- Date the prescription was issued and filled
- NDC number of the controlled substance dispensed
- Quantity of controlled substance dispensed
- Pharmacy's prescription number
- Pharmacy's DPS registration number

Emergency Dispensing a Schedule II

- Orally communicated prescription from a practitioner (in person or over telephone)
- Pharmacist must write down the prescription and include all the information required
  - For a standard prescription
  - For an official Schedule II prescription
- After dispensing, the pharmacist is responsible to
  - Maintain the written record/prescription created
  - Note the emergency nature of the prescription
  - Attach the original official prescription to the written record/prescription that was created
  - Retain both documents in the pharmacy records
  - Send the information required to the DPS
- Prescriber must send a written prescription within 7 days (or postmarked by the 7th day)
- Pharmacist must notify DEA office if the prescriber has not sent the written prescription

Partial Filling a Schedule II

- Can be for a written or emergency oral prescription
- Must have the quantity supplied written on the face of the prescription

- Must have the remaining balance filled within 72 hours of the first partial filling
- If cannot be filled within 72 hours: pharmacist must notify the prescriber and new prescription required (in other words, the prescription is now void)

Partial Filling a Schedule II for a Long-Term Care Facility (LTCF) or for a Terminally Ill Patient

- Must have "terminally ill" or "LTCF patient" on the face of the prescription
- For each partial filling, the dispensing pharmacist shall record on the back of the official prescription form:
    - date of the partial filling
    - quantity dispensed
    - remaining quantity authorized to be dispensed
    - identification of the dispensing pharmacist
- Total quantity dispensed cannot be more than the total quantity prescribed
- Prescription is valid for 60 days from date of issue

Faxed Schedule II Prescriptions

- Only valid for
    - Schedule II narcotic or non-narcotic LCTF patient and prescriber writes "LTCF patient" on Rx
    - Schedule II narcotic to be compounded for administration via parenteral, intravenous, intramuscular, subcutaneous, or intraspinal infusion
    - Schedule II narcotic for a terminally ill or hospice patient with "terminally ill" or "hospice patient" on Rx
    - After faxing, the prescriber should

- o Write "VOID – sent by fax to (name and telephone number of receiving pharmacy)" on the prescription
- o File the prescription with the patient's medical records

Section Five: Texas Controlled Substance Laws Regarding Schedule III–V's

- Anabolic steroids and human growth hormone are Schedule III
- Need to ID people picking up controlled prescriptions if not known to the pharmacist
- Must be a valid patient-practitioner relationship
- May be refilled up to 5 times within the 6-month period after date of issuance
- Must have DPS number of provider on every prescription
  (if provider licensed in Texas)
- May fill a prescription from an out of state practitioner IF practitioner is authorized by the other state to prescribe the substance

Prescription Requirements

Controlled substance prescription must contain:
- Date of issue
- Name and address of the patient
  - If an animal, the species of the animal and the name and address of its owner
- Name of the controlled substance prescribed
- Quantity (Arabic numeral followed by the number written as a word)
- Directions for use
- Intended use of the drug unless the practitioner determines that information to not be in the best interest of the patient

- Manual signature of the prescriber
- Prescriber's
    o legibly printed or stamped name
    o address
    o DEA number
    o telephone number

Dispensing an Emergency Quantity upon Discharge

May dispense a Schedule III–V to a patient that is admitted to a hospital** and will require an emergency quantity upon release
- Properly labeled container
- May be an amount as determined appropriate by the attending practitioner as needed for proper treatment of the patient until the patient can obtain access to a pharmacy
- **Hospital* –a general hospital, special hospital, licensed ambulatory surgical center, surgical suite in a dental school, or veterinary medical school
    o May refer to a hospital clinic or emergency room, if the clinic or emergency room is under the control, direction, and administration as an integral part of a general or special hospital

Submitting Prescription Information to DPS

Must submit to the DPS no later than the 15th day after the last day of the month in which the prescription is completely filled
- Practitioner's DPS number (unless out of state)
- Patient's (or the animal owner's name) name, age (or date of birth)
- Patient's address (including city, state, and ZIP code)
- Date prescription issued and filled
- NDC number of the controlled substance dispensed

- Quantity of controlled substance dispensed
- Pharmacy's prescription number
- Pharmacy's DPS registration number

Records

Keep all records for a minimum of 2 years from the latest date when
- Record was required to be created
- Record was actually created
- Prescription was last filled

Emergency Refills

- May be done **in case of**
  - Interruption of drug regimen
  - Patient suffering
  - Natural/manmade disaster preventing contact with prescriber
  - Inability to make contact the prescriber after reasonable effort
- Quantity must not exceed 72-hour supply
  - Inform patient that it is being provided without authorization and that patient must see prescriber for future refills
  - Inform prescriber of the emergency refill at earliest reasonable time
- Emergency dispensing in a natural/manmade disaster
  - Max of 30-day supply
  - No Schedule IIs
  - Allowed only if all apply:
    - Interruption of regimen
    - Patient suffering
    - Disaster prevents contact with prescriber

- Governor has declared state of disaster
- Texas State Board of Pharmacy notifies pharmacies they may dispense up to a 30-day supply

Delivery of Controlled Substances

May deliver a controlled substance by an authorized delivery person, a person known to the pharmacist, a pharmacist intern, by the authorized delivery person, or by mail

- Maintain the following record for at least 2 years
- Name of the authorized delivery person
- Name of the person known to the pharmacist, pharmacist intern, or authorized delivery person
- Mailing address to where delivery is made, if being mailed

Designated Agents

- A designated agent must be one of the following:
  - Registered nurse licensed in Texas
  - Licensed vocational nurse licensed in Texas
  - Physician assistant licensed in Texas
  - Employee who is:
    - located in the practitioner's office **and**
    - a member of the health care staff of the office
- A practitioner must maintain in the practitioner's usual place of business a current written list of each individual designated as an agent under this section

Inspection

May not examine, audit, inspect, inventory, or copy without consent:
- financial data
- sales data (other than shipment data)
- pricing data

Discrepancies/Theft

- Must notify the director of DPS not later than the **third** day after the date the person learns of:
    - Discrepancy in the amount of an item ordered from the amount received
    - Loss or theft during shipment or from current inventory
- Not later than close of business **on the day of discovery**, a practitioner must report a lost or stolen official prescription form to **both**:
    - Local police department or sheriff's office
    - Director of the Texas Prescription Program

Section Six: Texas Pharmacy Act

Purpose
The purpose of this legislation is to promote, preserve, and protect the public health, safety, and welfare through:
- effectively controlling and regulating the practice of pharmacy
- licensing pharmacies engaged in the sale, delivery, or distribution of prescription drugs and devices used in diagnosing and treating injury, illness, and disease

The Texas State Board of Pharmacy
- Consists of 11 members appointed by the governor with approval by the senate
  - 7 members – pharmacists
  - 3 members – public
  - 1 member – pharmacy technician
- There must be pharmacists employed in Class A and Class C pharmacies
- An appointed pharmacist board member must be
  - Resident of Texas
  - Licensed for the previous 5 years
  - Licensed in good standing
  - Practicing pharmacy in Texas
- An appointed pharmacy technician board member must be
  - Resident of Texas
  - Registered for the previous 5 years
  - Registration in good standing
  - Be an acting pharmacy technician in Texas
- A potential public board member is ineligible if the person or the person's spouse
  - Works in health care (example: licensed)

- o Owns a business (>10% interest) that is regulated by the board
- o Directly receives goods/services/money from the board
- o Works/manages a business that receives funds from the board
- A person may not be a member of the board if a
  - o Registered lobbyist
  - o Person or person's spouse works for a Texas trade association in the field of health care
- Terms are 6 years
  - o If vacancy during term, governor appoints replacement
  - o No more than 2 consecutive full terms
- Governor appoints president of the board
- Board elects other officers

Board Inspections
Board may inspect
- Drug storage and security
- Equipment
- Compounding materials
- Sanitary conditions
- Records

Board may **not** inspect
- Financial data
- Sales data
- Pricing data

Dispensing
- On the prescription (the hard copy) the pharmacist will write
  - o Drug name
  - o Drug strength

- o Drug manufacturer
- Label requirements
  - o Brand name
    - ▪ if no brand name, then generic name, strength, and manufacturer of drug
  - o Name, address, and telephone number of pharmacy
  - o Date prescription dispensed
  - o Name of prescriber
  - o Name of patient
    - ▪ if for an animal, then species of animal and name of owner
  - o Instructions for use
  - o Quantity dispensed
  - o The date after which the drug must not be used (if not in an original container)
- Labeling requirements do not apply to an inmate being released if the prescription is no more than a 10-day supply

Substitution
- Generic substitution must have the words "substituted for brand prescribed" or "substituted for [brand name]" where [brand name] = brand name of the drug prescribed
- Pharmacist may not select a generically equivalent drug unless it costs the patient less than the prescribed drug
- If the drug costs < patient copay, then must charge for the price of the drug
- Must be a valid practitioner-patient relationship in order to dispense a prescription
  - o Internet-based or telephonic consultation is not allowed
  - o May dispense in an emergency (physician covering the office's pager)
- Pharmacist may change the dosage form (tablet instead of capsule, liquid instead of tablet) if
  - o Contains identical amount of active ingredients

- o Not enteric-coated or timed-release product
- o Does not alter desired clinical outcomes

Narrow Therapeutic Index Drugs

- List developed by the Texas Medical Board and Board of Pharmacy
- May only be refilled using the same drug product and manufacturer
- If same drug product by same manufacturer not available, may dispense a generically equivalent drug
  - o Must notify the patient when prescription dispensed
  - o Must notify the prescriber no later than 72 hours after dispensing
- May not interchange immunosuppressant drug (ex: generic for brand) without *prior* consent from prescriber
- If prescriber is unavailable, then
  - o Notify and receive consent from the patient
  - o Notify prescriber no later than 24 hours after dispensing

Rules for Different Classes of Pharmacies

- Class A or Class B – requires continuous on-site supervision of a pharmacist during business hours for pharmacy services
- Class C with >100 beds – requires continuous on-site supervision of a pharmacist during business hours for pharmacy services
- Class C with < 100 beds – requires pharmacist present part-time or on a consulting basis
- Class D – requires continuous supervision of a pharmacist whose services are required according to the needs of the pharmacy

- Class E – requires continuous on-site supervision of a pharmacist and requires a pharmacist-in-charge

Rural Hospital Rules
- Definition – licensed hospital with ≤ 75 beds
  - In a county with ≤ 50,000 people; **or**
  - Designated by the Centers for Medicare and Medicaid Services as a critical access hospital, rural referral center, or sole community hospital
- If pharmacist not on duty – nurse or practitioner may withdraw drug/device from the pharmacy or from floor stock
- Pharmacist will verify withdrawal and perform drug regimen review not later than 7th day after withdrawal
- If a pharmacy technician is registered with the board; and a pharmacist is accessible at all times; and a nurse, practitioner, or a pharmacist can verify the accuracy of the technician via remote access – then they may do the following without direct supervision of a pharmacist:
  - Enter medication orders
  - Prepare, package, or label a prescription if a licensed nurse or practitioner verifies the accuracy prior to administration
  - Fill a medication cart
  - Distribute stock supplies to patient care areas
  - Restock automated medication supply cabinets
  - Perform any other duty specified by board rule

Automated Pharmacy System
- Definition – mechanical system that dispenses prescription drugs and maintains the transaction records

- Class A or C pharmacy may use an automated pharmacy system in a facility not at the same location as the Class A or C pharmacy
- Pharmacist in charge of Class A or C pharmacy is responsible for filling and loading the storage containers for medication stored in bulk at the facility
- Automated pharmacy system must be under continuous supervision by a pharmacist
  - Can be done electronically (pharmacist doesn't have to be physically present)
- Automated system is only allowed at a health care facility regulated by the state

Telepharmacy System

- Definition – system that monitors the dispensing of prescription drugs and provides for related drug use review and patient counseling services by an electronic method, including the use of the following types of technology:
  - audio and video
  - still-image capture
  - store and forward
- Class A or C pharmacies in Texas may use this system to dispense drugs in a facility that is not at the same location
- Must be under continuous supervision of a pharmacist
  - Is not required to be physically present
  - May supervise electronically through audio and video communication
- Must be located at a health care facility in Texas
- May not have a Class A or C pharmacy in the same community as the telepharmacy system
- If a Class A or C pharmacy opens in the community, the telepharmacy system can continue to be used

Compounding Rules
- Office use – supplying a compounded drug for administration by a practitioner for a patient in a treatment setting
- Prepackaging – repacking and relabeling drugs into unit dose packaging or a multiple dose container for distribution
- May dispense a compounded drug for office use by a practitioner
- Must comply with US Pharmacopoeia guidelines when compounding
- May advertise/promote
  - Non-sterile prescription compounding services
  - Specific compounded drug products

Dispensing of Dangerous Drugs in Certain Rural Areas
- Reimbursement for cost – an additional charge by the physician that includes drug product and other actual costs to the physician in order to dispense. Does not include a separate fee for actually dispensing the drug
- Certain rural areas – county ≤5,000 population or municipality or an unincorporated town ≤2,500 population that is within a 15-mile radius of the physician's office and where a pharmacy is not located
- Does not apply if located next to a municipality ≥2,500 population
- A physician may
  - Maintain a supply of dangerous drugs
  - Dispense these drugs in the course of treating patients

- Be reimbursed for the cost of supplying the drugs without obtaining a license
- The physician must
  - Comply with labeling provisions and make sure in compliance with packaging and record keeping
  - Notify the pharmacy board and the Texas State Board of Medical Examiners

Veterinarians
- May administer or provide dangerous drugs to a patient in their office
- May delegate the administration to a qualified and trained person
- Receive compensation for the drugs
- May not maintain a pharmacy for selling drugs—must have a license
- Must comply with laws relating to the practice of veterinary medicine and state and federal laws relating to dangerous drugs

Manufacturer Label Requirements
- Name and business address of the original manufacturer of the finished dosage form
- Name and business address of each repackager or distributor of the drug before delivery to pharmacist
- Does not apply to a distributor that only acts as a wholesaler and does not repackage or modify drug packages

Section Seven: Texas Dangerous Drug Act

- Keep prescription 2 years after date of initial dispensing or last refilling — whichever is later
- Against the law to possess dangerous drugs except in the usual course of business or practice by (or an agent/employee of) the following:
  - Licensed pharmacy
  - Practitioner
  - Person who performs lawful research, teaching, or testing
  - Hospital for administration by a practitioner
  - Officer/employee of the federal, state, or local government
  - Licensed manufacturer or wholesaler
  - Carrier or warehouseman
  - Licensed home and community support services agency
  - Licensed midwife who obtains oxygen for administration to a mother or newborn or who obtains a dangerous drug for the administration of prophylaxis to a newborn for the prevention of ophthalmia neonatorum
  - Licensed salvage broker or salvage operator
  - Certified laser hair removal professional
- Refilling a dangerous drug without authorization is allowed when
  - Therapeutic regimen is interrupted
  - Patient is suffering
  - Disaster prevents contact with prescriber
  - Pharmacy is unable to contact prescriber
  - Quantity does not exceed 72-hour supply

- After unauthorized refill, pharmacist must
    - Notify patient that being provided without authorization
    - Notify prescriber as soon as possible

Section Eight: Texas Administrative Code

Grounds for Discipline for a Pharmacist License

"Unprofessional conduct" is defined as engaging in behavior or committing an act that fails to conform with the standards of the pharmacy profession, including but not limited to, criminal activity or activity involving moral turpitude, dishonesty, or corruption. This conduct shall include, but not be limited to:

- Dispensing a prescription drug pursuant to a forged, altered, or fraudulent prescription
- Dispensing a prescription drug order pursuant to a prescription from a practitioner as follows:
  - Dispensing of a prescription drug order not issued for a legitimate medical purpose or in the usual course of professional practice shall include the following:
    - Dispensing controlled substances or dangerous drugs to an individual or individuals in quantities, dosages, or for periods of time which grossly exceed standards of practice, approved labeling of the federal food and drug administration, or the guidelines published in professional literature; or
    - Dispensing controlled substances or dangerous drugs when the pharmacist knows or reasonably should know that the controlled substances or dangerous drugs are not necessary or required for the patient's valid medical needs or for a valid therapeutic purpose

- Delivering or offering to deliver a prescription drug or device in violation of this act, the controlled substances act, the dangerous drug act, or rules promulgated pursuant to these acts
- Acquiring or possessing or attempting to acquire or possess prescription drugs in violation of this act, the controlled substances act, the dangerous drug act, or rules adopted pursuant to these acts
- Distributing prescription drugs or devices to a practitioner or a pharmacy not in the course of professional practice or in violation of this act, the controlled substances act, dangerous drug act, or rules adopted pursuant to these acts
- Refusing or failing to keep, maintain, or furnish any record, notification, or information required by this act, the controlled substances act, dangerous drug act, or any rule adopted pursuant to these acts
- Refusing an entry into any pharmacy for any inspection authorized by the act
- Making false or fraudulent claims to third parties for reimbursement for pharmacy services
- Operating a pharmacy in an unsanitary manner
- Making false or fraudulent claims concerning any drug
- Persistently and flagrantly overcharging for the dispensing of controlled substances
- Dispensing controlled substances or dangerous drugs in a manner not consistent with public health or welfare
- Failing to practice pharmacy in an acceptable manner consistent with public health and welfare
- Refilling a prescription upon which there is authorized "PRN" refills or words of similar meaning, for a period of time in excess of one (1) year from the date of issuance of such prescription
- Engaging in any act, acting in concert with another, or engaging in any conspiracy resulting in a restraint of

trade, coercion, or a monopoly in the practice of pharmacy
- Sharing or offering to share with a practitioner compensation received from an individual provided pharmacy services by a pharmacist
- Obstructing a board employee in the lawful performance of his duties of enforcing the act
- Engaging in conduct that subverts or attempts to subvert any examination or examination process required for a license to practice pharmacy. Conduct that subverts or attempts to subvert the pharmacist licensing examination process includes, but is not limited to:
    - Copying, retaining, repeating, or transmitting in any manner the questions contained in any examination administered by the board or questions contained in a question pool of any examination administered by the board
    - Copying or attempting to copy another candidate's answers to any questions on any examination required for a license to practice pharmacy
    - Obtaining or attempting to obtain confidential examination materials compiled by testing services or the board
    - Impersonating or acting as a proxy for another in any examination required for a license to practice pharmacy
    - Requesting or allowing another to impersonate or act as a proxy in any examination required for a license to practice pharmacy; or
    - Violating or attempting to violate the security of examination materials or the examination process in any manner

- Violating the provisions of an agreed board order or board order
- Dispensing a prescription drug while not acting in the usual course of professional pharmacy practice
- Failing to provide or providing false or fraudulent information on any application, notification, or other document required under this act, the dangerous drug act, the controlled substances act, or rules adopted pursuant to those acts
- Physically abusing a board employee during the performance of such employees lawful duties
- Failing to establish or maintain effective controls against the diversion or loss of controlled substances or dangerous drugs, loss of controlled substance or dangerous drug records, or failure to ensure that controlled substances or dangerous drugs are dispensed in compliance with state and federal laws or rules, by a pharmacist who is:
  - A pharmacist-in-charge of a pharmacy
  - A sole proprietor or individual owner of a pharmacy
  - A partner in the ownership of a pharmacy; or
  - A managing officer of a corporation, association, or joint-stock company owning a pharmacy.
    - A pharmacist is equally responsible with an individual designated as pharmacist-in-charge of such pharmacy to ensure that employee pharmacists and the pharmacy are in compliance with all state and federal laws or rules relating to controlled substances or dangerous drugs
- Failure to respond within the time specified on a warning notice issued as a result of a compliance inspection

- Responding to a warning notice as a result of a compliance inspection in a manner that is false or misleading
- Being the subject of civil fines imposed by a federal or state court as a result of violating the controlled substances act or dangerous drug act
- The sale, purchase, or trade—or the offer to sell, purchase, or trade—of prescription drug samples; however, this paragraph does **not** apply to:
    - Prescription drugs provided by a manufacturer as starter prescriptions or as replacement for such manufacturer's outdated drugs
    - Prescription drugs provided by a manufacturer in replacement for such manufacturer's drugs that were dispensed pursuant to written starter prescriptions; **or**
    - Prescription drug samples possessed by a pharmacy or a health care entity which provides health care primarily to indigent or low-income patients at no or reduced cost — **if**:
        - The samples are possessed in compliance with the prescription drug marketing act of 1987
        - The pharmacy is owned by a charity or by a city, state, or county government; **and**
        - The samples are for dispensing or provision at no charge to patients of that health care entity.
- The sale, purchase, or trade—or the offer to sell, purchase, or trade—of prescription drugs:
    - Sold for export use only
    - Purchased by a public or private hospital or other health care entity; **or**
    - Donated or supplied at a reduced price to a charitable organization

- The above 3 points do not apply to:
  - The purchase or other acquisition by a hospital or other health care entity which is a member of a group purchasing organization, or from other hospitals or health care entities which are members of such an organization;
  - The sale, purchase, or trade of a drug or an offer to sell, purchase, or trade a drug by an organization to a nonprofit affiliate of the organization to the extent otherwise permitted by law
  - The sale, purchase, or trade of a drug or an offer to sell, purchase, or trade a drug among hospitals or other health care entities which are under common control
  - The sale, purchase, or trade of a drug—or an offer to sell, purchase, or trade a drug—for emergency medical reasons, including the transfer of a drug between pharmacies to alleviate temporary shortages of the drug arising from delays in or interruptions of regular distribution schedules
  - The dispensing of a prescription drug pursuant to a valid prescription drug order to the extent otherwise permitted by law;
- The sale, purchase, or trade—or the offer to sell, purchase, or trade—of:
  - Misbranded prescription drugs; **or**
  - Prescription drugs beyond the manufacturer's expiration date
- Failure to repay a guaranteed student loan

- Failure to respond and to provide all requested records within the time specified in an audit of continuing education records under the title relating to Continuing Education Requirements
- Allowing an individual whose license to practice pharmacy, either as a pharmacist or a pharmacist-intern, or a pharmacy technician/trainee whose registration has been disciplined by the board, resulting in the license or registration being revoked, canceled, retired, surrendered, denied, or suspended, to have access to prescription drugs in a pharamcy

Grounds for Discipline for a Pharmacy License

A pharmacy fails to establish and maintain effective controls against diversion of prescription drugs when
- There is inadequate security or procedures to prevent unauthorized access to prescription drugs; **or**
- There is inadequate security or procedures to prevent the diversion of prescription drugs

Grounds for discipline for a pharmacy license
- During the time an individual's license to practice pharmacy, either as a pharmacist or a pharmacist-intern, or a pharmacy technician's registration has been disciplined by the board, resulting in the license or registration being revoked, canceled, retired, surrendered, denied, or suspended, the pharmacy employs or allows such individual access to prescription drugs;
- The pharmacy possesses or engages in the sale, purchase, or trade—or the offer to sell, purchase, or trade—prescription drug samples;

- The pharmacy possesses or engages in the sale, purchase, or trade—or the offer to sell, purchase, or trade—of prescription drugs
  - Sold for export use only
  - Purchased by a public or private hospital or other health care entity; **or**
  - Donated or supplied at a reduced price to a charitable organization and possessed by a pharmacy other than one owned by the charitable organization;
- The pharmacy engages in the sale, purchase, or trade— or the offer to sell, purchase, or trade—of
  - Misbranded prescription drugs; **or**
  - Prescription drugs beyond the manufacturer's expiration date
- The owner or managing officer has previously been disciplined by the board

Grounds for Discipline for a Pharmacy Technician or a Pharmacy Technician Trainee

"Negligent, unreasonable, or inappropriate conduct" shall include, but not be limited to:
- Delivering or offering to deliver a prescription drug or device in violation of the Controlled Substances Act, the Dangerous Drug Act, or rules promulgated pursuant to these Acts
- Acquiring or possessing or attempting to acquire or possess prescription drugs in violation of this Act, the Controlled Substances Act, the Dangerous Drug Act, or rules adopted pursuant to these Acts
- Failing to perform the duties of a pharmacy technician or pharmacy technician trainee in an acceptable manner consistent with the public health and welfare, which

contributes to a prescription not being dispensed or delivered accurately
- Obstructing a board employee in the lawful performance of his duties of enforcing the Act
- Violating the provisions of an agreed board order or board order, including accessing prescription drugs with a revoked or suspended pharmacy technician or pharmacy technician trainee registration
- Physically abusing a board employee during the performance of such employees lawful duties
- Failing to repay a guaranteed student loan

Denial of a License
- If an original application or request for renewal of a license is denied, then can make a written request within 30 days for a hearing

Reporting Professional Liability Claims
- Duty to report
  - If insured, then the insurance provider reports to the board
  - If uninsured, then the license holder must report
- Report within 30 days after receiving the notice of claim letter or complaint

Out of State Disciplinary Actions
For disciplinary actions taken by a regulatory board of another state, the board has determined the following shall be applicable for all types of licensees and registrants for such licenses and registrations issued by the board

- If the other state's disciplinary action resulted in the license or registration being restricted, suspended, revoked, or surrendered, the appropriate sanction shall be the same as the sanction imposed by the other state, such that the licensee or registrant has the same restriction against practice in Texas
- If the license or registration is subject to any other type of disciplinary sanctions, the appropriate sanction shall be equivalent to or less than that imposed by the other state unless contrary to board policy
- The sanctions opposed by this section can be used in conjunction with other types of disciplinary actions including administrative penalties

Section Nine: Pharmacists

- Pharmacist-in-charge is responsible for ensuring that the pharmacy is in compliance with all state and federal laws and rules
- All pharmacists while on-duty are responsible for complying with all state and federal laws and rules
- Register with the board every 2 years (biennially)
- Must publicly display the pharmacist's license and license renewal certificate in the pharmacist's primary place of practice
- May not call yourself a pharmacist unless licensed as a pharmacist
- Notify board within 10 days of change of address, name, or place of employment

Requirements to be a Licensed Pharmacist
- At least 18 years old
- Good moral character
- Minimum 1,500-hour internship. Obtain hours through one of the following:
    - Board approved student internship program
    - Board approved extended-internship program
    - Graduate from college/school of pharmacy after July 1, 2007 and will be credited 1,500 hours or the number of hours actually obtained and reported by the college
    - Internship hours approved and certified to the board by another state board of pharamcy
- Graduated from an accredited pharmacy program

- Passed the required examinations
  (if fail – may retake twice)
- If licensed in another state – must be/have been in good standing

Reciprocity Requirements
- Pay fee
- Complete application under oath
- Good moral character
- Graduated from accredited pharmacy degree program
- Proof of current/initial licensing by exam
- Proof of current license being in good standing
- Pass the Texas MPJE
- Cannot reciprocate unless other state grants reciprocal licensing under similar conditions
- Cannot practice pharmacy with an expired license

Emergency Temporary Pharmacist License
- In an emergency situation, the board may grant a pharmacist who holds a license to practice pharmacy in another state an emergency temporary pharmacist license to practice in Texas
- Applicant must have a license in another state that is in good standing and be sponsored by a pharmacy in Texas with an active license
- Emergency temporary pharmacist license is only valid for a time period set by the board or up to 6 months

Pharmacist License Renewal
- License expires on last day of the expiration month

- If renewal application and fee not received on or by the last day of the assigned expiration month, then the license will expire
- Cannot practice pharmacy with an expired license
- Expired license by 90 days or less – pay 1.5 times the renewal fee
- Expired license by more than 90 days – pay 2 times the renewal fee
- Expired license by 1 year or more – apply for new license

Continuing Education Requirements

- Must complete 30 hours every two years
- For renewals received after January 1, 2014, at least one contact hour must be related to Texas pharmacy laws or rules
- Obtaining CE
  - Complete the continuing education hours
  - Pass the NAPLEX, which is equivalent to 30 hours
  - Have a Texas pharmacist license issued by examination or reciprocity within the previous 24 months
- Exempt from continuing education requirements during initial license period
- Many ways to earn CE, such as BCLS, ACLS, PALS, and attending a Texas State Board of Pharmacy Board Meeting (3 hours – max of 6 hours during a license period)
- Receive 3 hours of CE for passing an initial Board of Pharmaceutical Specialties certification examination
- May receive credit for completing programs approved by the American Medical Association as Category 1 Continuing Medical Education (CME)

- May receive credit for programs or courses approved by other boards of pharmacy
- Keep CE records (hard copy or electronic format) for 3 years from date of reporting them on a license renewal application – may be audited!

Placing a License on Inactive Status
- Currently licensed
  - Failed to complete CE requirements
  - Not practicing in Texas
- Cannot practice if license is inactive
- Making an inactive license active
  - Fill out form
  - Complete CE requirements (up to 30 hours)

Licenses for Military Spouses
Applicant for pharmacist's license who is the spouse of a person serving on active duty as a member of the armed forces of the United States
- Reciprocity
  - May be granted a temporary license prior to completing the NABP application and taking and passing the Texas MPJE
    - Complete application
    - Meet the educational and age requirements
    - Present proof of initial licensing by examination and proof that current license and any other licenses have not been suspended, revoked, canceled, surrendered or otherwise restricted for any reason
    - Submit fingerprints and criminal background check

- Pay licensing fee
- Provide documentation that spouse is active duty military such as marriage certificate and military identification
- Expired Texas pharmacist's license
  - License expired within 5 years preceding the application date and the applicant lived in another state for at least 6 months
    - Complete application
    - Provide documentation that spouse is active duty military such as marriage certificate and military identification
    - Pay renewal fee
    - Complete approved continuing education
      - Expired 1-2 years then complete 15 hours
      - Expired 2-3 years then complete 30 hours
      - Expired 3-5 years then complete 45 hours
    - Not required to take Texas MPJE
- These temporary pharmacist licenses are valid for 6 months only and may be extended only by board approval
- Temporary license expires within 6 months if individual fails to pass the Texas MPJE within 6 months or fails to take the Texas MPJE within 6 months
- Cannot serve as a pharmacist in charge of a pharmacy with a temporary pharmacist license

Failing an Exam

If an applicant passes the Texas Pharmacy Jurisprudence Exam but fails NAPLEX, the applicant may use the passing grade on the Jurisprudence examination for licensure purposes for a period of two (2) years from the date of passing the exam.

Section Ten: Pharmacist-Interns

Hours

- 1,500 hours of internship required for licensure
- Maximum of 50 hours per week may be counted
- Internship hours expire 2 years after internship completed
- Hours can be earned in another state if they are approved and certified by another state board of pharmacy

Student-Intern Requirements

- Must register with the board before beginning an internship
- Must notify board within 10 days for change of address or name
- Must do all of the following:
  - Submit an application to the board
  - Enroll in an ACPE accredited program
  - Complete first professional year with a minimum of 30 credit hours of course work
  - Run a criminal background check, including fingerprints

Student-Intern Card

- Expires when any of the following apply:
  - Cease enrollment in school
  - Fail the NAPLEX® and/or MPJE® examinations
  - Fail to take the NAPLEX® and/or MPJE® within 6 calendar months after graduation

- Board may extend the extend the student internship if the NAPLEX® or MPJE® are suspended or delayed

Pharmacist-Intern Identification

- Board will provide documentation that authorizes the individual to perform the duties of a pharmacist-intern
- Pharmacist-intern must keep that written documentation with them at all times while acting as a pharmacist-intern
- Pharmacist-intern must wear an identification badge that lists their name and status as a pharmacist-intern

Intern Duties

A student-intern or extended-intern may perform any duty of a pharmacist, provided the duties are delegated by and under the supervision of a pharmacist licensed by the board and approved as a preceptor by the board

- Initiating and receiving refill authorization requests
- Entering prescription data into the computer
- Taking a stock bottle from the shelf
- Preparing and packaging prescription drug orders (e.g., counting tablets and placing them in the prescription container)
- Affixing prescription labels and auxiliary labels
- Reconstituting medication
- Prepackaging and labeling prepackaged drugs
- Loading bulk unlabeled drugs into an automated dispensing system, provided a pharmacist verifies the system is properly loaded prior to use
- Bulk compounding

- Compounding non-sterile preparations, provided the intern has completed the pharmacist training requirements
- Compounding sterile preparations, provided the intern has completed the pharmacist training requirements
- Administering immunizations, provided the intern has completed the pharmacist training requirements

When not under the supervision of a pharmacist preceptor, the intern may function as a pharmacy technician without having to register as a pharmacy technician with the board, provided the intern

- Registered as a pharmacist-intern with the board
- Is under the direct supervision of a pharmacist
- Completed the on-site pharmacy technician training
- Is not counted in the ratio of pharmacists to pharmacy technicians
    - ratio of pharmacists to interns when the intern is functioning as a technician is 1:1

Pharmacist-Interns May Not

- Present or identify himself/herself as a pharmacist
- Sign or initial any document which is required to be signed by a pharmacist, unless the preceptor cosigns
- Independently supervise pharmacy technicians or trainees

Extended-Intern

- Considered an extended-intern provided one of the following requirements are met:
    - Passed NAPLEX and Texas MPJE but lack internship hours for licensure

- Applied to the board to take NAPLEX and Texas MPJE within 6 calendar months after graduation and has:
  - Graduated and received a professional degree from a college/school of pharmacy; or
  - Completed all the requirements for graduation and receipt of a processional degree from a college/school of pharmacy
- Applied to the board to take the NAPLEX and Texas MPJE within 6 calendar months after obtaining full certification from the Foreign Pharmacy Graduate Equivalency Commission
- Applied to the board for re-issuance of a pharmacist license which has expired for more than 2 years but less than 10 years and has successfully passed the Texas MPJE but lacks the internship hours or continuing education required for licensure
- Resident in a residency program accredited by the American Society of Health-System Pharmacists in the state of Texas
- Ordered by the board to complete an internship
- Internship must be board approved and in a pharmacy licensed by the board, or a federal government pharmacy
- Must be in the presence of and under the direct supervision of a pharmacist preceptor
- Effective for two years but expires immediately when
  - Failure to take NAPLEX or Texas MPJE within 6 calendar months after graduation or FPGEC certification
  - Failure to pass the NAPLEX and Texas MPJE
  - Upon termination of the residency program
  - Obtaining a pharmacist license

Section Eleven: Preceptors

Requirements
- Either
  - A pharmacist currently licensed by the board and not on inactive status
  - A healthcare professional preceptor
- Pharmacist preceptor must display the pharmacist preceptor certificate with their license and their renewal certificate

Pharmacist Preceptor Requirements
- At least
  - One (1) year as a licensed pharmacist; **or**
  - 6 months of residency training in an ASHP accredited program
- Complete 3 hours of pharmacist preceptor training approved by the ACPE
- To maintain certification, 3 hours of approved pharmacist preceptor training is required in the current pharmacist license renewal period

Ratios
- Pharmacist to intern ratio may only be 1:1 **unless** supervision is part of a Texas college/school of pharmacy program; then there is no ratio requirement

Section Twelve: Drug Therapy Management

Drug Therapy Management

Definition – the performance of specific acts by pharmacists as authorized by a physician through written protocol. May include:
- collecting and reviewing patient drug use histories
- ordering or performing routine drug therapy–related patient assessment procedures including temperature, pulse, and respiration
- ordering drug therapy–related laboratory tests
- implementing or modifying drug therapy following diagnosis, initial patient assessment, and ordering of drug therapy by a physician as detailed in the protocol; **or**
- any other drug therapy–related act delegated by a physician

Written Protocol

Definition – a physician's order, standing medical order, standing delegation order, or other order or protocol as defined by rule of the Texas Medical Board under the Medical Practice Act. Must at minimum:
- identify the individual physician authorized to prescribe drugs and responsible for the delegation of drug therapy management
- identify the individual pharmacist authorized to dispense drugs and to engage in drug therapy management as delegated by the physician

- identify the types of drug therapy management decisions that the pharmacist is authorized to make, which shall include:
  - ailments or diseases involved, drugs, and types of drug therapy management authorized; **and**
  - procedures, decision criteria, or plan the pharmacist will follow when exercising drug therapy management authority
- state the activities the pharmacist will follow in the course of exercising drug therapy management authority, including the method for documenting the decisions made and a plan for communication or feedback to the authorizing physician concerning specific decisions made. Documentation shall be recorded within a reasonable time of each intervention and may be performed on the patient medication record, patient medical chart, or in a separate log book; **and**
- describe appropriate mechanisms and time schedule for the pharmacist to report to the physician monitoring the pharmacist's exercise of delegated drug therapy management and the results of the drug therapy management

Performing Drug Therapy Management

A pharmacist may perform drug therapy management (implementation or modification of a patient's drug therapy under a protocol – including authority to sign a prescription drug order for dangerous drugs) provided all of the following conditions are met:

- Physician must first diagnose, perform an initial patient assessment and start drug therapy

- Pharmacist must practice in a hospital, hospital-based clinic, or an academic health care institution that has bylaws and a medical staff policy that permits a physician to delegate to a pharmacist

Signing Prescriptions

Pharmacist who signs prescriptions for dangerous drugs must
- Notify the board that a physician has delegated the authority
  - Fill out board application
  - Occur prior to signing any prescriptions
  - Updated annually
  - Include a copy of the written protocol
- On each prescription
  - Pharmacist's name, address, and telephone number
  - Delegating physician's name, address and telephone number

Board Will Post on its Website

- Name and license number of each pharmacist allowed to sign prescriptions
- Name and address of delegating physician
- Expiration date of the protocol

Pharmacist Training Requirements

- At least 6 hours of CE related to drug therapy each year

Physician Requirements

- Formulates or approves the written protocol

- Establishes and maintains a physician-patient relationship with each patient
- Physically present each day
- Receives a periodic status report on each patient on a schedule defined in the protocol
- Available for direct telecommunication
- Makes sure pharmacist maintains a pharmacist-patient relationship with each patient

Records

- All records must be kept for at least two (2) years from date of record

Written Protocol

- Pharmacist must keep a copy of the written protocol and any patient-specific deviations
- Pharmacist documents all interventions
- Physician and pharmacist must annually review and document the written protocol

Section Thirteen: Administration of Immunizations or Vaccinations

Written Protocol

- A physician's order, standing medical order, or standing delegation order must contain, at minimum, the following:
    - Prescribing physician
    - Administering pharmacist
    - Location of administration (address)
    - Vaccines that will be administered
    - Actions the pharmacist will follow in administering vaccines
    - Reporting procedures
    - Standard protocol may be used or may have patient specific deviations

Pharmacist Certification Requirements

- BCLS – must be maintained/in date
- Evidence-based course – one-time course
    - Study material
    - Hands-on training for administering vaccines
    - Testing with a passing score
    - Meets CDC training guidelines
    - Minimum of 20 hours of instruction and experiential training
- Continuing education – 3 hours of CE every 2 years on disease states, drugs, and administration of vaccines

Supervision by Physician

- Established physician-patient relationship required with each patient under 14 years old, except a pharmacist may administer the influenza vaccine to a patient over 7 years old
- Prescriber must be geographically located to be easily accessible to the pharmacist
- Receives periodic status reports on patients
- Available for direct telecommunication

Special Provisions

- Pharmacists can only administer vaccines under a written protocol
- Patient that is under 14 years old – can only administer upon referral from a physician who has an established physician-patient relationship
- Influenza vaccine may be administered to patients over the age of 7 without an established physician-patient relationship
- May administer vaccines within a pharmacy or any other location identified in the written protocol
- May **not** be administered where the patient resides, except for a licensed nursing home or hospital
- Authority of a pharmacist to administer vaccines may not be delegated

Notifications

- Pharmacist that administers vaccines will provide notification of administration to both
  - Physician in the written protocol within 24 hours of administration

- Primary care physician of the patient within 14 days of administration
- Notification will include
    - Name and address of patient
    - Age of patient (if under 14)
    - Name of patient's primary care physician
    - Name, manufacturer, and lot number of vaccine administered
    - Amount administered
    - Date administered
    - Site of administration
    - Route of administration
    - Name, address, and title of the person administering the vaccine

Records

- Keep for 2 years
- Include everything listed above in Notifications

Section Fourteen: Pharmacy Technicians

Pharmacy Technicians

- Only allowed to do non-judgmental technical duties under direct supervision by a pharmacist
- May receive license discipline from the board just like a pharmacist's license

Registration Requirements

- Must register with the board to be employed or perform the duties of a pharmacy technician or pharmacy technician trainee
- If registered previously as a technician, then can't register as a trainee
- Must publically display current registration certification in primary place of employment
- Must notify board within 10 days of change of name, address, or employment

Pharmacy Technician Trainee

- May only register once and will not be renewed
- Must register with the board before beginning work
- Requires
    - High school diploma/GED or will achieve in 2 years
    - Application
    - Criminal history
- Expires two (2) years from date of registration or when registered as a pharmacy technician

Registration Requirements

- Have a high school diploma (or GED) or working towards one for no more than 2 years
- Must have either
  - Passed the PTCB examination
  - Been granted exemption
- Complete application
- Pay fee

Exemption from PTCB Examination

Petition for exemption from certification requirement if
- Live in a county with population <50,000; **or**
- Have been employed as a pharmacy technician in Texas for at least 10 years and employer approves the petition (as of 9/1/01)

Registration Renewal

- Requirements
  - Complete application
  - Pay fee
  - Complete 20 hours of CE
- Expires on last day of assigned expiration month
- Cannot work with an expired registration
- Register every 2 years

Continuing Education

- Trainees – not required
- First time technician registered – Not required in initial registration period
- Maximum of 10 hours can be earned at workplace
- One hour must be pharmacy law
- Keep records for 3 years

Tech-Check-Tech

- Allowed if Class C pharmacy has an ongoing clinical pharmacy program
- Allows a pharmacy technician to verify the accuracy of work performed by another pharmacy technician relating to the filling of floor stock and unit dose distribution systems for a patient admitted to the hospital, if the patient's orders have previously been reviewed and approved by a pharmacist
- Must notify the board prior to beginning
- Pharmacist-in-charge of clinical pharmacy program makes the policies and procedures

Registration for Military Spouses – Alternative Registration Procedure

An applicant for a pharmacy technician registration who is the spouse of a person serving on active duty as a member of the armed forces of the United States may complete the following alternative procedures for registering as a pharmacy technician

- An applicant who held a pharmacy technician registration in Texas that expired within the five years preceding the application date and the registration expired while the applicant lived in another state for at least six months who meets the following requirements may be granted a pharmacy technician registration. The applicant:
  - Shall complete the Texas application for registration that includes the following:
    - Name
    - Addresses, phone numbers, date of birth, and social security number; however, if an individual is unable to obtain a social security number, an individual taxpayer identification number may be provided in

lieu of a social security number along with documentation indicating why the individual is unable to obtain a social security number
- Any other information requested on the application
- Shall provide documentation that the applicant is the spouse of a member of the armed forces of the United States to include:
  - Marriage certificate; and
  - Military identification indicating that the:
    - Applicant is a military dependent; and
    - Applicant's spouse is on active duty status
- Pay the registration fee
- Criminal history check including fingerprints
- Not required to have a current PTCB certificate

Registration for Military Spouses – Expedited Registration Procedure

An applicant for a pharmacy technician registration who is the spouse of a person serving on active duty as a member of the armed forces of the United States and who holds a current registration as a pharmacy technician issued by another state may complete the following expedited procedures for registering as a pharmacy technician. The applicant shall:
- Have a high school or equivalent diploma (e.g., GED), or be working to achieve a high school or equivalent diploma. For the purpose of this clause, an applicant for registration may be working to achieve a high school or equivalent diploma for no more than two years; and
- Have taken and passed the Pharmacy Technician Certification Board's National Pharmacy Technician Certification Examination or other examination

94

approved by the board and have a current certification certificate; and

- Complete the Texas application for registration that includes the following information:
  - o Name
  - o Addresses, phone numbers, date of birth, and social security number; however, if an individual is unable to obtain a social security number, an individual taxpayer identification number may be provided in lieu of a social security number along with documentation indicating why the individual is unable to obtain a social security number; and
  - o Any other information requested on the application
- Meet all requirements necessary in order for the Board to access the criminal history record information, including submitting fingerprint information and paying the required fees; and
- Pay the registration fee

Section Fifteen: Destruction of Dispensed Drugs

Returning Unused Dangerous Drugs
- Pharmacist practicing/consulting in a health care facility, or a licensed health care professional that administers drugs in a jail **may** return dangerous drugs (not controls) **if**
    - Medications are individually packaged; **and**
    - Medication is not subject to recall by state/federal agency or manufacturer
- Pharmacist practicing/consulting in a health care facility, or a licensed health care professional that administers drugs in a jail **may not** return a drug
    - Has been compounded
    - Appears to be adulterated
    - Requires refrigeration
    - Has <120 days until expiration date
- Pharmacy may restock and redistribute these returned drugs and must credit Medicaid

Drugs Dispensed to Patients in Healthcare Facilities
By a consultant pharmacist
- Only dangerous drugs
- A consultant pharmacist may not destroy controlled substances unless allowed to do so by federal laws or rules of the DEA
- Written agreement between facility and consultant
- Inventoried

- o Name and address of facility
- o Name and license number of consultant pharmacist
- o Date of drug destruction
- o Date the prescription was dispensed
- o Prescription number
- o Name of dispensing pharmacy
- o Name, strength, quantity of drug
- o Signature of consultant pharmacist
- o Signature of witness(es)
- o Method of destruction
- Must be destroyed to render the drugs unfit for human consumption
- Must be witnessed by one of the following:
  - o Commissioned peace officer
  - o Agent of the board
  - o Agent of the THHSC
  - o Agent of the Texas Department of State Health Services
  - o Any two of the following:
    - Facility administrator
    - Director of nursing
    - Acting director of nursing
    - Licensed nurse

Destruction of Drugs Dispensed to Patients in Healthcare Facilities by a Waste Disposal Service

A consultant pharmacist may utilize a waste disposal service to destroy dangerous drugs dispensed to patients in health care facilities or institutions. A consultant pharmacist may **not** use a waste disposal service to destroy controlled substances unless allowed to do so by federal laws or rules of the Drug Enforcement Administration. Dangerous drugs may be transferred to a waste disposal service for destruction.

Destruction by a Waste Disposal Service

- Only dangerous drugs
- Inventoried
  - Name and address of facility
  - Name and license number of consultant pharmacist
  - Date of packaging and sealing of the container
  - Date the prescription was dispensed
  - Prescription number
  - Name of dispensing pharmacy
  - Name, strength, and quantity of drug
  - Signature of consultant pharmacist packaging and sealing the container
  - Signature of the witness(es)
- Consultant pharmacist seals the container in presence of facility administrator and the director of nursing **or** one of the previously listed witnesses
- Waste disposal service will provide the facility with proof of destruction of the sealed container
  - Date, location, and method of destruction of the container and shall be attached to the inventory record

Dangerous Drugs Returned to a Pharmacy

- Drugs previously dispensed to a patient may be returned to the pharmacy
- No controls unless allowed by the DEA
- Destruction must make it unfit for human consumption
- Documentation must be kept
  - Name and address of dispensing pharmacy
  - Prescription number

- o Name and strength of dangerous drug
- o Signature of the pharmacist

Disposal of Stock Prescription Drugs

- Stock – in original manufacturer's container
- Pharmacist is allowed to destroy stock dangerous drugs
  - o Nalbuphine, and carisoprodol must be inventoried and destruction witnessed by another licensed pharmacist or a commissioned peace officer

Destruction of Stock Controlled Substances

- Two ways to destroy controlled substances
  1. Transfer to a disposal firm
  2. Destroy yourself with prior DEA approval
- Class A pharmacies – one (1) time per year
  - o Inventory and fill out DEA Form 41
  - o Send Form 41 to DEA at least 14 days in advance of destruction
    - no response = approval
  - o Must be destroyed beyond reclamation and witnessed by one of the following:
    - Commissioned peace officer
    - DEA agent
    - DPS agent
    - Board of Pharmacy agent
  - o Mail completed DEA Form 41 to DEA office
- Class C pharmacies
  - o Must obtain written authorization from DEA prior to destruction
  - o Inventory and fill out DEA Form 41

- o Destroy beyond reclamation, witnessed by one of the following:
    - Commissioned peace officer
    - Supervisory member of the hospital's security department
    - DEA agent
    - DPS agent
    - Board of Pharmacy agent
- o Mail completed DEA Form 41 to DEA office

Section Sixteen: Substitution of Drug Products

Generic Substitution

- May dispense a generically equivalent drug if
  - Generic drug costs less
  - Patient does not refuse
  - Prescriber does not certify brand medically necessary

Prohibiting Generic Substitution

- Prescriber must *handwrite* on the face of the prescription "brand necessary" or "brand medically necessary"
- When one form contains multiple prescription orders, prescriber must clearly specify which drug to which the directive applies, otherwise the pharmacist may substitute on all prescriptions on the form
- If a generic product becomes available, the pharmacist may substitute on refills unless doctor wrote "brand medically necessary" on the initial prescription
- Two-line prescription forms, check boxes, or other notations on an original prescription drug order which indicate "substitution instructions" are not valid methods to prohibit substitution, and a pharmacist may substitute on these types of written prescriptions
- For verbal and electronic prescriptions – prescriber may specify brand only and pharmacist cannot substitute

- The above statements do not apply to out-of-state prescriptions or to Mexican, Canadian, or federal facility practitioners

Patient Notification

- Before delivery of a prescription for a generically equivalent drug products, a pharmacist must
  - Inform patient a generically equivalent drug is available at a lower cost and ask the patient to choose between brand and generic
  - Display a sign in a prominent place in both English and Spanish: "TEXAS LAW REQUIRES A PHARMACIST TO INFORM YOU IF A LESS EXPENSIVE GENERICALLY EQUIVALENT DRUG IS AVAILABLE FOR CERTAIN BRAND NAME DRUGS AND TO ASK YOU TO CHOOSE BETWEEN THE GENERIC AND THE BRAND NAME DRUG. YOU HAVE A RIGHT TO ACCEPT OR REFUSE THE GENERICALLY EQUIVALENT DRUG."
  - If the cost of the drug is lower than the co-payment – must offer the lower price
  - Exceptions – patient authorization not needed on refills

Records

- Documentation required on the original/hard-copy prescription
  - Any substitution instructions communicated orally by the prescriber
  - Name and strength of actual drug product dispensed
    - Brand name and strength; **or**

- - Generic name, strength, and name of the manufacturer
- Refilled using a different manufacturer than previously dispensed – must provide the above information on the prescription
- NDC numbers may be used, but the above information must be documented

Determining Generic Equivalency
- Orange Book – "A" rating (AA, AB, AN, AO, etc.)
- Professional judgment

Section Seventeen: Laws Regarding Pharmacies

Display Requirements

- Cannot use the following terms unless a licensed pharmacy:
  - Pharmacy
  - Apothecary
  - Any graphic representation that implies pharmacy
- Must display the pharmacy license in full public view
- Class A or Class C that serves the public
  - Display the word "pharmacy" or a similar word or symbol as determined by the board in a prominent place on the front of the pharmacy; and
  - Display in public view the license of each pharmacist employed

Required Notifications to the Board

- Change of location or name – within 10 days
  - Send in license
  - Receive an amended one from the board
- Change of managing officers (top 4 executives) – within 10 days
- Change of ownership – License issued to previous owner must be returned to the board
- Change of employment – pharmacist notifies the board within 10 days

- Change of pharmacist-in-charge – within 10 days
  - Must do an inventory
- Loss/Theft – immediately upon discovery
  - Include a list of all controlled substances stolen or lost
- Fire/Disaster – within 10 days
- Keep all notifications for two (2) years

Closing a Pharmacy

- 14 days prior to closing
  - Notify DEA if have controlled substances
  - Post a sign notifying date of closing and acquiring pharmacy's information
- Closing day
  - Perform inventory
  - Transfer or destroy prescription drugs
  - Transfer patient files
  - Remove "pharmacy" from any signage
- After closing
  - Notify board (within 10 days of closing): date of closing, license, statement saying inventory done and how drugs transferred/destroyed, acquiring pharmacy's information
  - Send to DEA: registration, unused order forms, copy of any 222 forms used to transfer Schedule IIs from the closed pharmacy
  - Send in DPS registration

Recalls

- Must remove drug from stock within 24 hours of receiving recall notice

Return of Prescription Drugs

- May not resell or re-dispense a drug or prescription after it was originally dispensed or sold
- Unused drugs from a health care facility or penal institution must be
  - Sealed in unopened tamper proof packaging
  - Not subject to a recall
  - Not have been in the physical possession of the patient it was intended for
- Health care facilities and penal institutions may not return drugs that
  - Have been compounded
  - Appear adultered
  - Require refrigeration
  - Have <120 days until expiration

Pick up of Prescriptions

- May only pick up prescriptions at the pharmacy where it was dispensed
- Exceptions
  - Mail
  - Delivery to prescriber's home or office
  - Delivery to patient's home or employment location
  - Delivery to health care facility where patient is confined

Samples

Pharmacies may not sell, purchase, trade, or possess drug samples unless **all** of the following conditions are met:

- Owned by a charitable organization as defined by the IRS or by the city, state, or county government

- Provides care to primarily low-income, indigent populations
- Samples are dispensed/provided at no cost

Inventory Requirements

- Pharmacist-in-charge responsible, but may delegate
- Keep inventory records separate from all other records
- Inventory must be signed by both the person taking the annual inventory and the pharmacist-in-charge and indicate the day and time. PIC must have the inventory notarized within 72 hours or three working days of the completed inventory. Required for:
  - Annual inventory
  - Change of ownership inventory
  - Closing inventory
- Must include count of
  - All controlled substances
  - Nalbuphine
  - Tramadol for any inventory taken after January 1, 2013
- Exact count of all Schedule II
- Estimate count of Schedule III, IV, V and dangerous drugs, unless container holds >1,000 dosage, in which case an exact count must be made
- 3 separate records to be filed separately
  - Schedule II
  - Schedule III, IV, and V
  - Dangerous drugs
- Perpetual inventory must be reconciled on date of inventory
- Class C pharmacies must keep a perpetual inventory of Schedule I and IIs
- New Class A, Class C, or Class F pharmacy will take inventory on opening day of business

- o All controlled substances
- o All dosage form containing nalbuphine
- o For any inventory taken after January 1, 2013, all dosage forms containing tramadol
- Annual inventory required of Class A, C and F pharmacies
  - o All controlled substances
  - o All dosage form containing nalbuphine
  - o For any inventory taken after January 1, 2013, all dosage forms containing tramadol
- Change of ownership inventory required of Class A, C and F pharmacies
  - o All controlled substances
  - o All dosage form containing nalbuphine
  - o For any inventory taken after January 1, 2013, all dosage forms containing tramadol
- Change of pharmacist-in-charge inventory required of Class A, C, and F after January 1, 2013
  - o All controlled substances
  - o All dosage forms containing:
    - ▪ Nalbuphine
    - ▪ Tramadol

Professional Responsibility of Pharmacists

- Don't need a valid patient-physician relationship when prescribing for the partner of an sexually transmitted disease or family members of a patient that has an illness determined by Center for Disease Control to be a pandemic

Section Eighteen: Class A Pharmacy Rules

Personnel
- Each Class A pharmacy must have a pharmacist-in-charge (PIC) employed full-time
- Only can be a PIC at one (1) pharmacy except when
  - Both pharmacies are not providing services at the same time
  - An emergency requires a PIC to work at two (2) pharmacies as long as works at least 10 hours a week in each location for no more than 30 consecutive days
- Pharmacists must directly supervise technicians

Pharmacist Duties
Duties only a pharmacist can perform
- Receive oral prescriptions and write them down
- Interpret prescription drug orders
- Select of drug products
- Perform final check of prescription drug
- Counsel the patient
- Maintain patient records
- Interpret patient records and perform drug regimen review
- Manage drug therapy per written protocol
- Verify that controlled substances listed on invoices are received by clearly recording his/her initials and date of receipt of the controlled substances

Pharmacy Technician/Trainee Duties

- May not do any of the duties listed in the "Pharmacist Duties"
- Pharmacists may delegate any nonjudgmental tasks to pharmacy technicians/trainees provided that
  - Pharmacist verifies the accuracy
  - Technicians/trainees under direct supervision of a pharmacist
  - Must be trained on the automated pharmacy dispensing system
- Pharmacy technician/trainee duties
  - Initiating and receiving refill authorizations
  - Entering prescription data
  - Taking a stock bottle from the shelf for a prescription
  - Preparing and packaging prescription drug orders such as counting tablets/capsules, measuring liquids or placing them in the prescription container
  - Affixing prescription labels and auxiliary labels
  - Reconstituting medications
  - Prepackaging and labeling prepackaged drugs
  - Loading bulk unlabeled drugs into an automated dispensing system as long as a pharmacist verifies the accuracy before use
  - Compounding sterile and non-sterile drug products
  - Bulk compounding

Technician Ratios

- Except as provided below, the ratio of on-site pharmacists to pharmacy technicians and pharmacy technician trainees may be 1:4, provided the pharmacist is on-site and at least one of the four is a pharmacy technician. The ratio of

114

pharmacists to pharmacy technician trainees may not exceed 1:3
- May have a ratio of pharmacist to technician/trainees of 1:5 provided
  - Class A pharmacy
  - Dispenses no more than 20 different medications
  - Does not produce sterile preparations
  - At least 4 are pharmacy technicians (not trainees)
  - Written policies and procedures in place for supervision of the technicians

Identification of Pharmacy Personnel

- Pharmacy personnel must wear a badge that states person's name and title
- Titles are pharmacy, pharmacy technician, certified pharmacy technician, pharmacy technician trainee and pharmacist intern

Operational Standards

- Class A pharmacy registers annually or biennially with the board
- Notify board within 10 days of
  - Change of ownership – must apply for a new and separate license
  - Change of location/name – must file for an amended license
  - Change in managing officers
  - Closing of pharmacy
- Separate license is required for each location
- Pharmacy must be kept clean and in an orderly fashion
- Sink with hot and cold running water is required, exclusive of restroom facilities

- Counseling area must maintain confidentiality
- Flammable materials must be kept in a designated area for storage of flammable materials as set by local and state fire laws

Security

- Locked by key, combination, etc. to prohibit unauthorized access when a pharmacist is not on-site
- If the prescription department is closed at any time when the rest of the facility is open, the prescription department must be physically or electronically secured. The security may be accomplished by means such as floor to ceiling walls; walls, partitions, or barriers at least 9 feet 6 inches high; electronically monitored motion detectors; pull-down sliders; or other systems or technologies that will secure the pharmacy from unauthorized entrance when the pharmacy is closed
- Key, combination, or other mechanical or electronic means of locking the pharmacy may not be duplicated without the authorization of the pharmacist-in-charge or owner
- At a minimum, the pharmacy must have a basic alarm system with off-site monitoring and perimeter and motion sensors. The pharmacy may have additional security by video surveillance camera systems
- Pharmacy must maintain written documentation of authorized individuals other than individuals employed by the pharmacy who accessed the prescription department when a pharmacist is not on-site

Temporary Absence of Pharmacist – On-Site

One pharmacist on duty – may leave the prescription department for short periods of time without closing the prescription department and removing the remaining personnel as long as

- At least one pharmacy technician remains in the prescription department
- Pharmacist remains on-site at the licensed location of the pharmacy and is immediately available
- Pharmacist believes that the security of the prescription department will be maintained in their absence
- Notice is posted that says the pharmacist is on a break and the time the pharmacist will return
- Techs may begin the processing of prescription drug orders but may not deliver them until the pharmacist checks them
- Upon return, the pharmacist will
  - Review drug regimen
  - Verify accuracy of technicians
- Techs/personnel may deliver a previously verified prescription to a patient while the pharmacist is away as long as the following is documented
  - Date of delivery
  - Prescription number
  - Patient's name
  - Patient's phone number
  - Signature of person picking up the prescription
- While pharmacist is away, a pharmacist intern will be considered a registered pharmacy technician and may only do pharmacy technician duties
- When two (2) or more pharmacists on duty, stagger breaks

Temporary Absence of a Pharmacist – Off-Site

- Prescription department must be secured while not under the continuous on-site supervision of a pharmacist
- Technicians cannot perform any duties of a pharmacy technician
- May use an automated storage and distribution device for pickup of a previously verified prescription
  - Notice is posted that says
    - Pharmacist is off-site and not present
    - No new prescriptions maybe prepared but previously verified prescriptions may be delivered
    - Date/time the pharmacist will return
  - Must maintain documentation of the absences of the pharmacist
  - Prescription department is locked and secured
- Agent of the pharmacist may deliver a previously verified prescription during short periods of time when a pharmacist is off-site
  - Short time may not exceed two consecutive hours in a 24 hour period
  - Notice posted – same as above
  - Must maintain documentation of the absences of the pharmacist
  - Prescription department is locked and secured

Patient Counseling

Pharmacist shall communicate to the patient/patient's agent information about the prescription drug

- Name and description of the drug
- Dosage form, dosage, route, duration of therapy

- Special directions and precautions for preparation, administration, and use by the patient
- Common severe side effects
- Techniques for self-monitoring of drug therapy
- Proper storage
- Refill information
- Action to be taken in the event of a missed dose

Counseling Must be Provided

- Each new prescription drug order
- Any prescription drug order dispensed by the pharmacy on the request of the patient/patient's agent
- Communicated orally whenever possible
- Documented by recording the name of the patient, date of the counseling, prescription number and the initials of the pharmacist who provided the counseling in the prescription-dispensing record on one of the following:
    - On the original hard-copy prescription provided the counseling pharmacist clearly records his or her initials on the prescription for the purpose of identifying who provided the counseling
    - In the pharmacy's data processing system
    - In an electronic logbook; **or**
    - In a hard-copy log
- Must also provide written information
    - Plain language designed for the consumer
    - Easily readable font size – no smaller then 10 point Times New Roman
    - Compounded product – information about the major active ingredients
    - Must contain the statement "Do not flush unused medications or pour down a sink or drain."

- Only pharmacists may verbally provide drug information and answer questions concerning prescription drugs
- Non-pharmacist personnel may not ask questions of a patient which are intended to screen and/or limit interaction with the pharmacist
- If a patient refuses counseling, then don't have to provide it – just document refusal
- Pharmacy personnel shall inform the patient when refilling a prescription that a pharmacist is available to discuss the prescription and provide information
- A pharmacy shall post a sign no smaller than 8.5 inches by 11 inches in clear public view at all locations in the pharmacy where a patient may pick up prescriptions. The sign shall contain the following statement in a font that is easily readable: "Do you have questions about your prescription? Ask the pharmacist." Such notification shall be in both English and Spanish
- Must have a current or updated patient prescription drug information reference text or leaflets available for the public

Drug Regimen Review

Pharmacist shall, prior to or at the time of dispensing a prescription drug order, review the patient's medication record for
- Known allergies
- Rational therapy contraindications
- Reasonable dose and route of administration
- Reasonable directions for use
- Duplication of therapy
- Drug-drug interactions
- Drug-food interactions

- Drug-disease interactions
- Adverse drug reactions
- Proper utilization, including overutilization or underutilization

Substitution of Dosage Form

May dispense a dosage form different from what prescribed (example: liquid instead of tablets) if
- Pharmacist notifies practitioner
- Contains identical amount of active ingredients
- Not time-released/enteric coated
- Does not alter clinical outcomes

Prescription Containers

- Must be dispensed in a child-resistant container unless
  - Patient/prescriber request
  - Product exempt from requirements of the Poison Prevention Packaging Act of 1970
- Prescription containers or closures shall not be re-used

Labeling Requirements on a Prescription to be Dispensed

- Name, address, and phone number of the pharmacy
- Prescription number
- Date dispensed
- Dispensing pharmacist's initials
- Name of prescribing practitioner
- If prescription signed by a pharmacist, the name of the pharmacist who signed the prescription for a dangerous drug under delegated authority of a physician

- Name of the patient
  (or species of the animal and name of the owner)
- Instructions for use
- Quantity dispensed
- Ancillary instructions
- If the prescription is for a Schedules II–IV controlled substance, the statement "Caution: Federal law prohibits the transfer of this drug to any person other than the patient for whom it was prescribed"
- Generic substitution must have the statement "Substituted for Brand Prescribed" or "Substituted for [Brand Name]" where [Brand Name] is the actual name of the brand name product prescribed
- Name and strength of the actual drug dispensed
  - Brand name or generic name and name of the manufacturer
- Date after which the prescription should not be used (beyond-use date) – shall be one year from the date the drug is dispensed or the manufacturer's expiration date, whichever is earlier
- The name of the patient's partner or family member is not required to be on the label of a drug prescribed for a partner for a sexually transmitted disease or for a patient's family members if the patient has an illness determined by the Centers for Disease Control and Prevention, the World Health Organization, or the Governor's office to be pandemic

Returning Undelivered Medication to Stock
- May not resell/re-dispense any prescription that has been originally dispensed
- Prescriptions that have not been picked up may be returned to pharmacy stock for dispensing

- Must not be mixed within the manufacturer's container
- Must be used as soon as possible and stored in the dispensing container
- Expiration date is one (1) year from dispensing date on the prescription label or the manufacturer's expiration date if dispensed in the manufacturer's original container
- Must be placed in a new container when being dispensed **or** relabeled if using manufacturer's original container

Equipment and Supplies
- Data processing system, including a printer
- Refrigerator
- Child-resistant, light-resistant, tight containers
- Prescription, poison, and other labels
- Metric-apothecary weight and measure conversion charts
- Library – may be physical or electronic
  - Texas Pharmacy Act and rules
  - Texas Dangerous Drug Act and rules
  - Texas Controlled Substances Act and rules
  - Federal Controlled Substances Act and rules
  - At least one from each of the following categories
    - Patient information reference or leaflets with are designed for the patient and must be available to the patient
    - Drug interactions
    - General information reference text (Facts and Comparisons, Clinical Pharmacology, AHFS, Remington's)
  - Basic antidote information

- The telephone number of the nearest Regional Poison Control Center

Drugs

- Outdated drugs shall be quarantined from the dispensing stock
- Schedule V controlled substances containing codeine, dihydrocodeine, or any of the salts of codeine or dihydrocodeine may not be distributed without a prescription drug order from a practitioner
- A pharmacist may distribute nonprescription Schedule V controlled substances which contain no more than 15 milligrams of opium per 29.5729 ml or per 28.35 Gm provided
  - Only by a pharmacist, but someone else may completed the transaction
  - Not more than 240 ml or 48 solid dosage units of any substance containing opium to the same purchaser in any given 48-hour period
  - Purchaser at least 18 years of age
  - Proof of age/identification
  - Record: name and address of purchaser, name and quantity of controlled substance purchased, date of each purchase, signature/initials of distributing pharmacist

Customized Patient Medication Packages – Med-Pak

- Label requirements
  - Name of patient
  - Prescription number for the med-pak and each prescription drug order in the pak

- Name, strength, physical description or identification, and total quantity of each drug product
- Directions for use and cautionary statements
- Storage instructions or cautionary statements required by the official compendia
- Name of the prescriber of each drug product
- Name, address, and telephone number of the pharmacy
- Beyond-use date (one (1) year from date dispensed or earliest manufacturer's expiration date – whichever is less)

Automated Compounding or Counting Devices and Systems

- Must calibrate and verify accuracy on routine basis
- Container shall be labeled with the brand name and strength; **or** generic name, strength, and manufacturer
- Records of loading bulk drugs
  - Name of the drug, strength, and dosage form
  - Manufacturer **or** distributor
  - Manufacturer's lot number
  - Expiration date
  - Date of loading
  - Name, initials, **or** electronic signature of the person loading the automated compounding or counting device
  - Signature or electronic signature of the responsible pharmacist

Automated Storage and Distribution Device

Used to deliver a previously verified prescription to a patient when the pharmacy is open or closed

- Used to deliver refills and not new prescriptions
- May not deliver controlled substances
- Drugs must be stored at proper temperatures
- Patient is given the option to use the system
- Patient has access to a pharmacist for questions at the pharmacy by a telephone that connects directly to another pharmacy
- Loaded only by a pharmacist or a pharmacy technician or a pharmacy technician trainee under the direction and direct supervision of a pharmacist
- Located within the pharmacy building so pharmacy staff have access to the device from within the prescription department and patients have access to the device from outside the prescription department
- May not be located on an outside wall of the pharmacy
- May not be accessible from a drive-thru
- Must record a digital image of person picking up the prescription

Maintenance of Records

- Every inventory or other record – kept by the pharmacy and at the pharmacy's licensed location and available for at least two (2) years and supplied by the pharmacy within 72 hours
- Schedule II records – maintained separately
- Schedule III–V records – maintained separately or readily retrievable (controlled substances shall be asterisked, red-lined, or in some other manner readily identifiable apart from all other items appearing on the record)

Prescriptions

- If pharmacist questions the accuracy or authenticity of the prescription drug order – verify the order with the practitioner prior to dispensing
- Must make sure it is a valid prescription – there must be a valid patient-practitioner relationship
- Valid patient-practitioner relationship not needed in an emergency situation (ex. practitioner taking calls for the patient's regular practitioner)
- Written dangerous drug prescription orders
  - Manually signed by the practitioner; **or**
  - Electronically signed using a system which electronically replicates the practitioner's manual signature provided
    - System requires the practitioner to authorize each use
    - Prescription is printed on paper that is designed to prevent unauthorized copying and to prevent erasure or modification
- Schedule II, III, IV or V prescription forms must be manually signed
- Schedule II must also be issued on an official prescription form
- Rubber stamped is not allowed
- Sign prescription as any other legal document or check
- Cannot be signed by a practitioner's agent

Prescription Drug Orders Written by Out of State Practitioners

- Dangerous drugs – may be dispensed in the same manner as prescription drug orders for dangerous drugs issued by practitioners in Texas

- Schedule II
  - Filled in compliance with a written plan approved by the DPS and board
  - Practitioner registered with DEA and allowed to prescribe Schedule II in their state
  - Must be dispensed by the end of the 21th day after the date the prescription was issued
- Schedule III–V
  - Practitioner registered with DEA and allowed to prescribe Schedule III–V in their state
  - Not dispensed/refilled more than 6 months from initial date and not refilled more than 5 times
  - If out of refills – a new prescription required

Prescriptions Written by Practitioners in Mexico or Canada

- Schedule II–V – not allowed
- Dangerous drugs – allowed
  - Must be an original written prescription
  - Out of refills – new written prescription required

Prescriptions Carried Out or Signed by an Advanced Practice Nurse, Physician Assistant, or Pharmacist

- Practitioner shall make a list of each advanced practice nurse or physician assistant authorized to carry out or sign a prescription drug order
- No Schedule II drugs may be prescribed

Verbal Prescriptions

- Can only be received by a pharmacist or pharmacist-intern
- Practitioner will make a list of those allowed to verbally communicate prescriptions
- No verbal prescriptions from Canadian or Mexican practitioners

Electronic Prescriptions for Dangerous Drugs

- May be transmitted by a practitioner or practitioner's designated agent
    - Directly to a pharmacy; or
    - Through the use of a data communication device as long as it remains confidential
- Practitioner shall designate in writing the name of each agent authorized by the practitioner to electronically transmit prescriptions. List shall be available to pharmacists at request.
- Pharmacist may dispense an electronic prescription drug order for a Schedule II, III, IV or V controlled substance
- Electronic prescriptions not allowed for dangerous drug or controlled substance issued by a practitioner licensed in Canada or Mexico unless also licensed in Texas

Electronic Prescriptions for Controlled Substances

- A pharmacist may only dispense an electronic prescription drug order for a Schedule II, III, IV, or V controlled substance in compliance with the federal and state laws and the rules of the DEA

Faxed Prescription Drug Orders

- May be done for dangerous drugs
- Schedule III-V prescriptions must be manually signed by the practitioner and not electronically signed using a system that electronically replicates the practitioner's manual signature on the prescription drug order
- Not allowed for dangerous drugs or controlled substances from practitioner licensed in the Dominion of Canada or the United Mexican States unless the practitioner is also licensed in Texas

Prescription Records

- Stored in numerical order
- Keep for two (2) years from date of filling or the date the last refill dispensed
- Maintained in three (3) separate files
  - Schedule II
  - Schedule III–V
  - Dangerous drugs and nonprescription drugs

Prescription Requirements

- Name of the patient – or species of animal and name of the owner
- Address of patient (required for controlled substances)
- Name, address and telephone number of practitioner at the their usual place of business, legibly printed or stamped
  - If for a controlled substance, the DEA number of the practitioner
- Name and strength of the drug
- Quantity prescribed numerically and if for a controlled substance

- - Numerically followed by the number written as a word, if the prescription is written
  - Numerically if the prescription is electronic
  - If the prescription is communicated orally or telephonically, as transcribed by the receiving pharmacist
- Directions for use
- Intended use, unless that information would not be in the best interest of the patient
- Date of issuance
- If faxed
  - A statement that indicates the prescription has been faxed
  - If transmitted by a designated agent, the full name of the designated agent
- If electronically transmitted
  - The date the prescription drug order was electronically transmitted to the pharmacy if different from the date of issuance
  - If transmitted by a designated agent, the full name of the designated agent
- If issued by an advanced practice nurse or physician assistant
  - Name, address, telephone number, and if the prescription is for a controlled substance, the DEA number of the supervising practitioner
  - Address and telephone number of the clinic where the prescription drug order was carried out or signed

Pharmacist Documentation on Prescriptions

On either the original hard-copy prescription or in the pharmacy's data processing system, pharmacist must include
- Unique prescription number

- Initials or identification code of the dispensing pharmacist
- Initials or identification code of the pharmacy technician or pharmacy technician trainee performing data entry of the prescription
- Quantity dispensed, if different from quantity prescribed
- Date of dispensing, if different from date of issue
- Brand name or manufacturer of the drug dispensed

Documentation of Consultation with Prescriber

When a pharmacist consults a prescriber the pharmacist shall document on the hard-copy or in the pharmacy's data processing system associated with the prescription such occurrences and shall include the following information:
- Date the prescriber was consulted
- Name of the person communicating the prescriber's instructions
- Any applicable information pertaining to the consultation
- Initials or identifying code of the pharmacist performing the consultation clearly recorded for the purpose of identifying the pharmacist who performed the consultation if on the information is recorded on the hard-copy prescription

Refills

- Dangerous drugs or nonprescription drugs – may not be refilled after one (1) year from the date written
- Schedules III–V – may not be refilled more than five (5) times or after six (6) months from the date written
- Refilling without authorization for Schedule III–V and dangerous drugs

- o Interruption of therapeutic regimen/patient suffering
- o Does not exceed a 72-hour supply
- o Patient notified prescription being provided without authorization
- o Pharmacist informs practitioner at earliest reasonable time
- o Pharmacist maintains record of the emergency refill
- o Labels the dispensing container
- o If prescription filled at another pharmacy, then pharmacist may use professional judgment in refilling, provided
  - Patient has the prescription container, label, receipt, or other documentation which contains the essential information
  - Unable to contact other pharmacy to transfer or there are no refills remaining
  - Meets criteria for emergency refill and follows all the above steps
- Natural/manmade disaster
  - o Unable to contact prescriber
  - o Interruption of regimen/patient suffering
  - o Not Schedule II
  - o Maximum 30-day supply
  - o Governor has declared a state of disaster
  - o Board has notified pharmacies that can dispense up to a 30-day supply
  - o Patient notified prescription being provided without authorization
  - o Pharmacist informs practitioner at earliest reasonable time
  - o Pharmacist maintains record of the emergency refill
  - o Labels the dispensing container

Auto-Refill Program

A program that automatically refills prescriptions that have existing refills available in order to improve patient compliance

- Notice given of program given to patient and patient must indicate they want to enroll and must document
- Patient can withdraw at any time
- Only for dangerous drugs, and schedule IV and V controlled substances. Schedule II and III controlled substances may not be dispensed by an auto-refill program
- As is required for all prescriptions, a drug regimen review shall be completed on all prescriptions filled as a result of the auto-refill program. Special attention shall be noted for drug regimen review warnings of duplication of therapy and all such conflicts shall be resolved with the prescribing practitioner prior to refilling the prescription

Dispensing 90-Day Supply

May dispense up to a 90-day supply of a dangerous drug when the prescription specifies the dispensing of a lesser amount followed by periodic refills if

- Total quantity dispensed does not exceed the total quantity authorized on the original prescription including refills
- Patient consents to up to a 90-day supply
- Physician notified
- Physician has not specified on the prescription that dispensing the prescription in an initial amount followed by periodic refills is medically necessary
- Dangerous drug is not a psychotropic drug used to treat mental or psychiatric conditions
- Patient is at least 18 years old

Transfers

- Schedule III–V – only allowed once
  - Pharmacies electronically sharing a real-time, online database may transfer up to the maximum refills permitted by law and the prescriber's authorization
- Dangerous drugs – without limit
- Communicated orally by telephone or via facsimile directly by a
  - Pharmacist to another pharmacist
  - Pharmacist to a student intern, extended intern, or resident intern
  - Student intern, extended intern, or resident intern to another pharmacist
- Both the original and the transferred prescription drug orders are maintained for a period of two years from the date of last refill
- The individual transferring the prescription drug order information shall ensure the following occurs:
  - Write the word "void" on the face of the invalidated prescription or the prescription is voided in the data processing system
  - The following information is recorded on the reverse of the invalidated prescription drug order or stored with the invalidated prescription drug order in the data processing system:
    - Name, address, and if a controlled substance, the DEA registration number of the pharmacy to which such prescription is transferred
    - Name of the individual receiving the prescription drug order information
    - Name of the individual transferring the prescription drug order information; and
    - Date of the transfer

- The individual receiving the transferred prescription drug order information shall ensure the following occurs:
    - Write the word "transfer" on the face of the prescription or the prescription record indicates the prescription was a transfer
    - The following information if recorded on the prescription drug order or is stored with the prescription drug order in the data processing system:
        - Original date of issuance and date of dispensing or receipt, if different from date of issuance
        - Original prescription number and the number of refills authorized on the original prescription drug order
        - Number of valid refills remaining and the date of last refill, if applicable
        - Name, address, and if a controlled substance, the DEA registration number of the pharmacy from which such prescription drug order information is transferred
        - Name of the individual transferring the prescription drug order information

- Both the individual transferring the prescription and the individual receiving the prescription must engage in confirmation of the prescription information by such means as:
    - The transferring individual faxes the hard copy prescription to the receiving individual; or
    - The receiving individual repeats the verbal information from the transferring individual and

the transferring individual verbally confirms that the repeated information is correct

- Pharmacies using a data processing system shall comply with the following:
  - Prescription drug orders may not be transferred by non-electronic means during periods of downtime except on consultation with and authorization by a prescribing practitioner; provided however, during downtime, a hard copy of a prescription drug order may be made available for informational purposes only, to the patient or a pharmacist, and the prescription may be read to a pharmacist by telephone
  - The original prescription drug order shall be invalidated in the data processing system for purposes of filling or refilling, but shall be maintained in the data processing system for refill history purposes
  - If the data processing system does not have the capacity to store all the information required, the pharmacist is required to record this information on the original or transferred prescription drug order
  - The data processing system shall have a mechanism to prohibit the transfer or refilling of controlled substance prescription drug orders that have been previously transferred
- Pharmacies electronically accessing the same prescription drug order records may electronically transfer prescription information if the following requirements are met
  - The original prescription is voided and the pharmacies' data processing systems shall store all the information required

- Pharmacies not owned by the same person may electronically access the same prescription drug order records, provided the owner, chief executive officer, or designee of each pharmacy signs an agreement allowing access to such prescription drug order records
- An electronic transfer between pharmacies may be initiated by a pharmacist intern, pharmacy technician, or pharmacy technician trainee acting under the direct supervision of a pharmacist
- An individual may not refuse to transfer original prescription information to another individual who is acting on behalf of a patient and who is making a request for this information as specified in this subsection. The transfer of original prescription information must be done in a timely manner

Data Processing Systems

- Must maintain a backup copy of information stored in the data processing system using disk, tape, or other electronic backup system and update this backup copy on a regular basis, at least monthly, to assure that data is not lost due to system failure
- Pharmacist-in-charge shall report to the board in writing any significant loss of information from the data processing system within ten (10) days of discovery of the loss
- Must produce a daily hard-copy printout of all original prescriptions dispensed and refilled
  - Keep controlled substance records readily retrievable from non-controls
    - Each individual pharmacist that dispenses will verify the data on the printout and

initial within seven (7) days from the date of dispensing
- May also maintain a log book that each pharmacist can sign saying that information entered into the data processing system was correct

Distribution of Controlled Substances

A pharmacy may distribute controlled substances to a practitioner, another pharmacy, or other registrant, without being registered

- Recipient is registered to dispense controlled substances
- Total number of dosage units may not exceed 5% of all controlled substances dispensed and distributed during the twelve (12) month period
- Schedule I and II
  - Receiver shall issue Copy 1 and Copy 2 of a DEA 222 form to the pharmacy
  - Pharmacy keeps Copy 1 and forwards Copy 2 to DEA office

Records

- **All** Records (including prescriptions and inventory)
  - Must be kept for at least 2 years
  - Must be supplied within 72 hours of request
- Schedule I and II records must be maintained separately
- Records of controlled substances listed in Schedules III–V, other than prescription drug orders, shall be maintained separately or readily retrievable from all other records of the pharmacy
- Permanent log of the initials or identification codes which will identify each pharmacist, pharmacy

technician, and pharmacy technician trainee by name performing data entry of prescription information will be kept and each code or initials will be unique to the individual

Licensing Requirements for Compounding Sterile Preparations

A community pharmacy engaged in the compounding of sterile preparations shall be designated as a Class A-S pharmacy. Effective June 1, 2014 a Class A pharmacy may not compound sterile preparations unless the pharmacy has applied for and obtained a Class A-S pharmacy license

- Register annually or biennially with the board on a pharmacy license application provided by the board. A Class A-S license may not be issued unless the pharmacy has been inspected by the board to ensure the pharmacy meets the requirements as specified in §291.133 of this title (relating to Pharmacies Compounding Sterile Preparations)
- May not renew a pharmacy license unless the pharmacy has been inspected by the board within the last renewal period
- Notify board within ten days of the change of ownership and apply for a new and separate license
- Notify board within ten days with changes location and/or name for an amended license
- Notify board within ten days with changes in managing officers
- Notify board within ten days of closing
- A separate license is required for each principal place of business and only one pharmacy license may be issued to a specific location

Section Nineteen: Class B – Nuclear Pharmacy Rules

Owner

- Owner is responsible for all administrative and operational functions of the pharmacy
- PIC may advise the owner on administrative and operational functions
- Responsible at a minimum for the following and if not a Texas licensed pharmacist then will consult with the PIC or another Texas licensed pharmacist
    - Establishment of policies and procedures for procurement of prescription drugs and devices
    - Reviewing and approving policies related to the automated pharmacy dispensing system
    - Providing the pharmacy with the necessary equipment and resources
    - Policies related to storage, maintenance and retrieval of records

Pharmacist-In-Charge

- Every nuclear pharmacy must have a PIC
- Must be employed on a full-time basis
- May be PIC to more than one Class B pharmacy if
    - Class B pharmacies not open simultaneously
    - During an emergency, up to 2 Class B pharmacies open simultaneously if the PIC works at least 10 hours per week in each pharmacy for no more than a period of 30 consecutive days

Qualifications of Nuclear Pharmacists

- Meet minimal standards of training and experience in the handling of radioactive materials in accordance with the requirements of the Texas Regulations for Control of Radiation of the Radiation Control Program, Texas Department of State Health Services
- Licensed pharmacist in Texas
- Training – either
  - Current board certification as a nuclear pharmacist; **or**
  - Completed 700 hours in a structured educational program
    - 200 hours didactic training
    - 500 hours supervised practical experience

Technician Ratios

- Ratio of authorized nuclear pharmacists to pharmacy technicians and pharmacy technician trainees may be 1:4, provided at least one of the four is a pharmacy technician and is trained in the handling of radioactive materials
- Ratio of authorized nuclear pharmacists to pharmacy technician trainees may not exceed 1:3

Library

- Current copies of the following:
  - Texas Pharmacy Act and rules
  - Texas Dangerous Drug Act and rules
  - Texas Controlled Substances Act and rules; **and**
  - Federal Controlled Substances Act and rules (or official publication describing the requirements of the Federal Controlled Substances Act and rules)

- Current or updated version of Chapter 797 of the USP/NF concerning Pharmacy Compounding Sterile Preparations and other USP chapters applicable to the practice (e.g., USP Chapter 823 Radiopharmaceuticals for Positron Emission Tomography - Compounding); and
- Minimum of one current or updated text dealing with nuclear medicine science

Section Twenty: Class C Institutional Pharmacy Rules

Pharmacist Requirements

- >101 beds = must have continuous on-site supervision by a pharmacist
- <100 beds = part-time or consulting pharmacist must be on-site at least once every 7 days
- Must have 24/7 access to a pharmacist – can be via a pager

Pharmacist-In-Charge (PIC)

- ≥101 beds = must have one (1) full-time PIC
- ≤100 beds = must have one (1) PIC that is at least consulting or employed part-time – can be PIC for no more than 3 facilities or 150 beds
- PIC may be in charge of 1 facility with 101 beds or more and 1 facility with 100 beds or fewer, provided the total number of beds does not exceed 150 beds

Pharmacist Duties

- Providing those acts or services necessary to provide pharmaceutical care
- Receiving, interpreting, and evaluating prescription drug orders, and reducing verbal medication orders to writing either manually or electronically
- Participating in drug and/or device selection as authorized by law, drug and/or device supplier

selection, drug administration, drug regimen review, or drug or drug-related research
- Performing a specific act of drug therapy management for a patient delegated to a pharmacist by a written protocol from a physician licensed in this state
- Accepting the responsibility for
  - Distributing prescription drugs and devices with drug components, pursuant to medication orders
  - Compounding and labeling of prescription drugs and devices with drug components
  - Storing of prescription drugs and devices with drug components properly and safely
  - Maintaining proper records for prescription drugs and devices with drug components

Technician Duties in a Facility with ≥101 Beds

Must have pharmacist physically present to supervise
- Pre-packing and labeling unit and multi-dose packages – pharmacist will do final check
- Preparing, packaging, compounding, or labeling prescription drugs – pharmacist will do final check
- Bulk compounding or batch preparation – pharmacist will do final check
- Distributing routine orders for stock supplies to patient care areas
- Entering medication orders into data processing system – pharmacist will do final check
- Loading unlabeled drugs into an automated compounding or counting device, provided a pharmacist supervises, verifying that the system was properly loaded prior to use
- Accessing automated medication supply systems after proper training on the use of the automated medication supply system

- Compounding non-sterile preparations pursuant to medication orders, provided the pharmacy technicians or pharmacy technician trainees have completed the training
- Compounding sterile preparations pursuant to medication orders, provided the pharmacy technicians or pharmacy technician trainees
    - Have completed the required training
    - Are supervised by a pharmacist who has completed the required training and who conducts in-process and final checks

Technician Duties in a Facility with ≤100 beds

Pharmacist must be physically present to supervise unless the pharmacy meets the requirements for a rural hospital and has been approved by the board

- Pre-packing and labeling unit and multiple dose packages – final check by pharmacist
- Bulk compounding or batch preparation provided a pharmacist supervises and conducts in-process and final checks
- Loading unlabeled drugs into an automated compounding or counting device, provided a pharmacist supervises, verifying that the system was properly loaded prior to use
- Compounding medium-risk and high-risk sterile preparations pursuant to medication orders, provided the pharmacy technicians or pharmacy technician trainees
    - Have completed the training
    - Are supervised by a pharmacist who has completed the training and who conducts in-process and final checks

Electronic supervision by a pharmacist
- Preparing, packaging, or labeling prescription drugs pursuant to medication orders, provided a pharmacist checks the preparation prior to distribution
- Distributing routine orders for stock supplies to patient care areas
- Entering medication order and drug distribution information into a data processing system, provided judgmental decisions are not required and a pharmacist checks the accuracy of the information entered into the system prior to releasing the order
- Accessing automated medication supply systems after proper training on the use of the automated medication supply system and demonstration of comprehensive knowledge of the written polices and procedures for its operation
- Compounding non-sterile preparations pursuant to medication orders provided the pharmacy technicians or pharmacy technician trainees have completed the training
- Compounding low-risk sterile preparations pursuant to medication orders, provided the pharmacy technicians or pharmacy technician trainees
  - Have completed the training
  - Are supervised by a pharmacist who has completed the training and who conducts in-process and final checks

Tech-Check-Tech

- Only facilities with an ongoing clinical pharmacy program may allow a pharmacy technician to verify the accuracy of the duties performed by another pharmacy technician

- o Must be a registered pharmacy technician and not a technician trainee
- o Must have completed the required training
- Duties allowed to be performed
  - o Filling medication carts
  - o Distributing routine orders for stock supplies to patient care areas
  - o Accessing and restocking automated medication supply systems
- The patient's orders have previously been reviewed and approved by a pharmacist
- A pharmacist is on-duty in the facility at all times that the pharmacy is open for pharmacy services.

Rural Hospitals

Technicians may perform certain duties when a pharmacist is not on-duty if

- Registered as a pharmacy technician
- A pharmacist is accessible at all times to respond to any questions and needs of the pharmacy technician or other hospital employees, by telephone, answering or paging service, e-mail, or any other system that makes a pharmacist immediately accessible
- The pharmacy is appropriately staffed to meet the needs of the pharmacy
- A nurse or practitioner at the rural hospital or a pharmacist through electronic supervision verifies the accuracy of the actions of the pharmacy technician

Duties that are allowed when pharmacist is not present are

- Entering medication order and drug distribution information into a data processing system
- Preparing, packaging, or labeling a prescription drug according to a medication order if a licensed nurse or

practitioner verifies the accuracy of the order before administration of the drug to the patient
- Filling a medication cart used in the rural hospital
- Distributing routine orders for stock supplies to patient care areas
- Accessing and restocking automated medication supply cabinets

Identification of Pharmacy Personnel

- Must wear a badge that states person's name and title
- Titles are pharmacy, pharmacy technician, certified pharmacy technician, pharmacy technician trainee, and pharmacist intern

Library

- Texas Pharmacy Act and rules
- Texas Dangerous Drug Act and rules
- Texas Controlled Substances Act and rules
- Federal Controlled Substances Act and rules
- At least one (1) from each of the following categories
  - Drug interactions
  - General information reference text (Facts and Comparisons, USPDI Volume I, Clinical Pharmacology, AHFS, Remington's)
  - Injectable drugs reference
- Basic antidote information
- The telephone number of the nearest Regional Poison Control Center
- Metric-apothecary weight and measure conversion charts

Removing Drugs When Pharmacy Closed

Places with a full-time pharmacist
- Quantities removed must be only for immediate therapeutic needs
- Licensed nurse or practitioner may remove
- Record of removal
    - Name of patient
    - Name of drug, strength, dosage form
    - Dose prescribed
    - Quantity taken
    - Time and date
    - Signature of person removing
- Pharmacist verify withdrawal and do drug regimen review within 72 hours of withdrawal

Places with part-time or consultant pharmacist
- Same rules as above
- Pharmacist must verify withdrawal and do drug regimen review within 7 days

Floor Stock

- Must be in original manufacturer's container or prepackaged container
- Only can be removed by a designated licensed nurse or practitioner
- Record of withdrawal must be kept
    - Name of drug, strength, and dosage form
    - Quantity removed
    - Location of floor stock
    - Date and time
    - Signature of person making the withdrawal
- Pharmacist verifies withdrawal within 7 days

Formulary

- Must have a formulary
- Must have the PIC or a pharmacist designated by the PIC be a full voting member of the pharmacy and therapeutics committee

Prepackaging Drugs to be Kept at Facility

Label on prepackaged drug must include
- Brand or generic name, strength, name of manufacturer
- Facility's unique lot number
- Expiration date
- Quantity of drug if greater than one

Records of prepackaged drug
- Name of the drug, strength, and dosage form
- Facility's unique lot number
- Manufacturer or distributor
- Manufacturer's lot number
- Expiration date
- Quantity per prepackaged unit
- Number of prepackaged units
- Date packaged
- Name, initials, or electronic signature of the pre-packer
- Name, initials, or electronic signature of the responsible pharmacist

Sterile Preparations Prepared Outside the Pharmacy

Requires a label to be affixed to the container
- Patient's name and location, if not immediately administered
- Name and amount of drug(s) added

- Name of the basic solution
- Name or identifying code of person who prepared admixture
- Expiration date of solution

Medication Orders

- Drugs may be given to patients in facilities only on the order of a practitioner. No change in the order for drugs may be made without the approval of a practitioner except as authorized by the practitioner (no verbal orders from nurses)
- Pharmacy technicians and pharmacy technician trainees may not receive verbal medication orders

Discharge Prescriptions

Medications packaged in unit-of-use containers — such as metered-dose inhalers, insulin pens, topical creams or ointments, or ophthalmic or otic preparations — that are administered to the patient during the time the patient was a patient in the hospital may be provided to the patient upon discharge, provided the pharmacy receives a discharge order and the product bears a label containing the following information:

- Name of the patient
- Name and strength of the medication
- Name of the prescribing or attending practitioner
- Directions for use
- Duration of therapy (if applicable)
- Name and telephone number of the pharmacy

Drug Regimen Review

Conducted on a prospective basis when a pharmacist is on duty, except for an emergency order, and on a retrospective basis when a pharmacist is not on duty

Dispensing Take Home Medications from the ER

Must be dispensed by a pharmacist if on duty, but if pharmacist is not on duty
- Must have a list of approved dangerous drugs and/or controlled substances allowed to be supplied
- May only be supplied in prepackaged quantities not to exceed a 72-hour supply in suitable containers and appropriately pre-labeled (including necessary auxiliary labels) by the institutional pharmacy
- At the time of delivery of the dangerous drugs and/or controlled substances, the practitioner or licensed nurse under the supervision of a practitioner shall appropriately complete the label with at least the following information:
  - Name, address, and phone number of the facility
  - Date supplied
  - Name of practitioner
  - Name of patient
  - Directions for use
  - Brand name and strength of the dangerous drug or controlled substance
    - if not brand name, then the generic name, strength, and the name of the manufacturer or distributor of the dangerous drug or controlled substance
  - Quantity supplied
  - Unique identification number
- The pharmacy must keep a perpetual record of dangerous drugs and/or controlled substances supplied

- Date supplied
- Practitioner's name
- Patient's name
- Brand name and strength of the dangerous drug or controlled substance
  - if not brand name, then the generic name, strength, and the name of the manufacturer or distributor of the dangerous drug or controlled substance
- Quantity supplied
- Unique identification number
- The pharmacist must verify the record at least once every 7 days

Dispensing Drugs to Radiology Outpatients

Must be dispensed by a pharmacist if on duty, but if pharmacist is not on duty

- Prescription drugs may only be supplied to patients who have been scheduled for an X-ray examination at the facility
- Must be a system of control and accountability for prescription drugs administered or supplied in place
- Must have an approved drug list
- Prescription drugs may only be supplied in prepackaged quantities in suitable containers and pre-labeled by the institutional pharmacy with the following information:
  - Name and address of the facility
  - Directions for use
  - Name and strength
    - if generic name, the name of the manufacturer/distributor of the prescription drug
  - Quantity

- o   Facility's lot number and expiration date
- o   Appropriate ancillary label(s)
- At the time of delivery of the prescription drug, the practitioner or practitioner's agent shall complete the label with the following information:
  - o   Date supplied
  - o   Name of physician
  - o   Name of patient
  - o   Unique identification number
- A perpetual record of prescription drugs supplied from the radiology department shall be maintained in the radiology department. Such records shall include the following:
  - o   Date supplied
  - o   Practitioner's name
  - o   Patient's name
  - o   Brand name and strength
    - ▪   If no brand name, then the generic name, strength, dosage form, and the name of the manufacturer/distributor
  - o   Quantity supplied
  - o   Unique identification number
- Pharmacist verifies the record at least once every seven (7) days

Automated Devices and Systems

- Must have a method to calibrate and verify the accuracy of the automated compounding or counting device and document the calibration and verification on a routine basis
- Loaded with unlabeled drugs only by a pharmacist or by pharmacy technicians or pharmacy technician trainees under the direction and direct supervision of a pharmacist

- Label of an automated compounding or counting device container shall indicate the brand name and strength of the drug; or if no brand name, then the generic name, strength, and name of the manufacturer or distributor
- Records of loading unlabeled drugs into an automated compounding or counting device shall be maintained to show the following:
  o Name of the drug, strength, and dosage form
  o Manufacturer or distributor
  o Manufacturer's lot number
  o Expiration date
  o Date of loading
  o Name, initials, or electronic signature of the person loading the automated compounding or counting device
  o Signature or electronic signature of the responsible pharmacist
- May not be used until a pharmacist verifies that the system is properly loaded and affixes signature to the record

Automated Medication Supply Systems Used for Storage and Recordkeeping of Medications Located Outside of the Pharmacy Department (Pyxis)

A pharmacy technician or pharmacy technician trainee **may** re-stock an automated medication supply system located outside of the pharmacy department with prescription drugs, provided:
- Prior to distribution of the prescription drugs, a pharmacist verifies that the prescription drugs pulled to stock the automated supply system match the list of

prescription drugs generated by the automated medication supply system; **or**

- All of the following occur:
  - o Prescription drugs to re-stock the system are labeled and verified with a machine readable product identifier, such as a barcode
  - o Either
    - ▪ The drugs are in tamper evident product packaging, packaged by an FDA registered repackager or manufacturer, that is shipped to the pharmacy; or
    - ▪ If any manipulation of the product occurs in the pharmacy prior to restocking, such as repackaging or extemporaneous compounding, the product must be checked by a pharmacist; and
  - o Quality assurance audits are conducted according to established policies and procedures to ensure accuracy of the process

Maintenance of Records

- Every inventory or other record required to be kept shall be:
  - o Kept by the institutional pharmacy and be available, for at least two (2) years from the date of such inventory or record, for inspecting and copying by the board or its representative, and to other authorized local, state, or federal law enforcement agencies; **and**
  - o Supplied by the pharmacy within 72 hours
- Records of controlled substances listed in Schedule I and II shall be maintained separately from all other records of the pharmacy

- Records of controlled substances listed in Schedules III–V shall be maintained separately or readily retrievable from all other records of the pharmacy.
    - "Readily retrievable" means that the controlled substances shall be asterisked, redlined, or in some other manner readily identifiable apart from all other items appearing on the record.
- Records, except when specifically required to be maintained in original or hard-copy form, may be maintained in an alternative data retention system, such as a data processing or direct imaging system, e.g., microfilm or microfiche, provided
    - Records in the alternative data retention system contain all of the information required on the manual record; **and**
    - Alternative data retention system is capable of producing a hard copy of the record upon the request of the board, its representative, or other authorized local, state, or federal law enforcement or regulatory agencies.

Outpatient Records
- Follow Class A rules
- Outpatient discharge prescriptions must be written as regular prescriptions – medication order forms or copies thereof do not meet the requirements for outpatient forms
- Controlled substances listed in Schedule II must be written on an official prescription form in accordance with the Texas Controlled Substances Act
- Outpatient prescriptions for Schedule II controlled substances that are exempted from the official prescription requirement must be manually signed by the practitioner.

Original Medication Orders

Each original medication order shall bear the following information:
- Patient name and room number or identification number
- Drug name, strength, and dosage form
- Directions for use
- Date
- Signature or electronic signature of the practitioner or that of his or her authorized agent

Original medication order shall be maintained with the medication administration records of the patients

Patient Medication Records (PMR)

A patient medication record shall be maintained for each patient of the facility. The PMR shall contain at a minimum the following information:
- Patient name and room number or identification number
- Gender and date of birth or age
- Weight and height
- Known drug sensitivities and allergies to drugs and/or foods
- Primary diagnoses and chronic conditions
- Primary physician
- Other drugs the patient is receiving

Loss of Data

The pharmacist-in-charge shall report to the board in writing any significant loss of information from the data processing system within 10 days of discovery of the loss

Distribution of Controlled Substances to Another Registrant

A pharmacy may distribute controlled substances to a practitioner, another pharmacy or other registrant, without being registered to distribute, under the following conditions:

- Registrant to whom the controlled substance is to be distributed is registered under the Controlled Substances Act to dispense that controlled substance
- Total number of dosage units of controlled substances distributed by a pharmacy may not exceed 5.0% of all controlled substances dispensed or distributed by the pharmacy during the 12-month period in which the pharmacy is registered
  - If at any time it does exceed 5%, the pharmacy is required to obtain an additional registration to distribute controlled substances

Schedule III, IV, or V controlled substances – a record shall be maintained which indicates

- Actual date of distribution
- Name, strength, and quantity of controlled substances distributed
- Name, address, and DEA registration number of the distributing pharmacy
- Name, address, and DEA registration number of the pharmacy, practitioner, or other registrant to whom the controlled substances are distributed

Schedule I or II controlled substances

- Receiver (pharmacy, practitioner or other registrant) shall issue Copy 1 and Copy 2 of a DEA order form (DEA 222) to the distributing pharmacy
- Distributing pharmacy shall
  - Complete the area on the DEA 222 titled *TO BE FILLED IN BY SUPPLIER*

- Maintain Copy 1 of the DEA 222 at the pharmacy for two years
- Forward Copy 2 of the DEA 222 to the divisional office of the Drug Enforcement Administration

Other Records to be Maintained by a Pharmacy

- Permanent log of the initials or identification codes that will identify pharmacy personnel by name
    - The initials or identification code shall be unique to ensure that each person can be identified (e.g., identical initials or identification codes cannot be used)
- Copy 3 of DEA order form (DEA 222), properly dated, initialed, and filed; and all copies of each unaccepted or defective order form and any attached statements or other documents
- Hard copy of the power of attorney to sign DEA 222 order forms
- Suppliers' invoices of dangerous drugs and controlled substances
    - A pharmacist shall verify that the controlled drugs listed on the invoices were actually received by clearly recording his/her initials and the actual date of receipt of the controlled substances
- Suppliers' credit memos for controlled substances and dangerous drugs
- Hard copy of inventories
    - Except a perpetual inventory of controlled substances listed in Schedule II may be kept in a data processing system if the data processing system is capable of producing a hard copy of the perpetual inventory on-site

- Hard copy reports of surrender or destruction of controlled substances and/or dangerous drugs to an appropriate state or federal agency
- Records of distribution of controlled substances and/or dangerous drugs to other pharmacies, practitioners, or registrants
- Hard copy of any notification required by the Texas Pharmacy Act or these sections, including—but not limited to—the following:
    - Reports of theft or significant loss of controlled substances to DEA, DPS, and the board
    - Notifications of a change in PIC of a pharmacy
    - Reports of a fire or other disaster that may affect the strength, purity, or labeling of drugs, medication, devices, or other materials used in diagnosis or treatment of injury, illness, and disease

Permission to Maintain Central Records

Any pharmacy that uses a centralized recordkeeping system for invoices and financial data
Controlled substances
- Submit written notification to the DEA and TSBP
- May maintain central records commencing 14 days after receipt of notification by the divisional director
- Shall not include executed DEA order forms, prescription drug orders, or controlled substance inventories, which shall be maintained at the pharmacy
Dangerous drug records
- Invoices and financial data for dangerous drugs may be maintained at a central location
- Must deliver records to the pharmacy location within 2 business days of written request

Compounding Sterile Preparations

Effective August 31, 2014, a Class C pharmacy shall not compound sterile preparations unless the pharmacy has applied for and obtained a Class C-S pharmacy

- Register annually or biennially
- Must be inspected by the board prior to receiving license
- Must be inspected by the board prior to renewing license
- If the Class C-S pharmacy is owned or operated by a hospital management or consulting firm, the following conditions apply:
    - The pharmacy license application shall list the hospital management or consulting firm as the owner or operator
    - The hospital management or consulting firm shall obtain DEA and DPS controlled substance registrations that are issued in their name, unless the following occurs:
        - The hospital management or consulting firm and the facility cosign a contractual pharmacy service agreement which assigns overall responsibility for controlled substances to the facility
        - Such hospital pharmacy management or consulting firm maintains dual responsibility for the controlled substances
- Notify board within 10 days of changing ownership and apply for new license
- Notify board within 10 days of changing location and/or name to receive an amended license
- Notify board within 10 days of changing managing partners
- Notify board within 10 days of closing

- A separate license is required for each principal place of business and only one pharmacy license may be issued to a specific location
- A Class C-S pharmacy with an ongoing clinical pharmacy program that proposes to allow a pharmacy technician to verify the accuracy of work performed by another pharmacy technician relating to the filling of floor stock and unit dose distribution systems for a patient admitted to the hospital if the patient's orders have previously been reviewed and approved by a pharmacist shall make application to the board as follows.
  - The pharmacist-in-charge must submit an application on a form provided by the board, containing the following information:
    - Name, address, and pharmacy license number
    - Name and license number of the pharmacist-in-charge
    - Name and registration numbers of the pharmacy technicians
    - Anticipated date the pharmacy plans to begin allowing a pharmacy technician to verify the accuracy of work performed by another pharmacy technician
    - Documentation that the pharmacy has an ongoing clinical pharmacy program
    - Any other information specified on the application
  - The pharmacy may not allow a pharmacy technician to check the work of another pharmacy technician until the board has reviewed and approved the application and issued an amended license to the pharmacy

- Every two years, in connection with the application for renewal of the pharmacy license, the pharmacy shall provide updated documentation that the pharmacy continues to have an ongoing clinical pharmacy program

Section Twenty-One: Class C Pharmacies Located in a Freestanding Ambulatory Surgical Center (ASC) Rules

Personnel

- Each ambulatory surgical center shall have one (1) PIC who is employed or under contract, at least on a consulting or part-time basis, but may be employed on a full-time basis
- The consultant pharmacist may be the PIC
- A written contract shall exist between the ASC and any consultant pharmacist, and a copy of the written contract shall be made available to the board upon request

Operational Standards

- The pharmacy must register annually with the board
- A separate license is required for each principal place of business
- Only one (1) pharmacy license may be issued to a specific location

Library

- Texas Pharmacy Act and rules
- Texas Dangerous Drug Act and rules
- Texas Controlled Substances Act and rules

- Federal Controlled Substances Act and rules **or** official publication describing the requirements of the Federal Controlled Substances Act and rules
- At least one current or updated reference from each of the following categories:
  o Drug interactions
  o General information
- A current or updated reference on injectable drug products, like *Handbook of Injectable Drugs*
- Basic antidote information and the telephone number of the nearest regional poison control center
- If the pharmacy compounds sterile preparations, specialty references appropriate for the scope of services provided by the pharmacy
  o E.g., if the pharmacy prepares cytotoxic drugs, a reference text on the preparation of cytotoxic drugs, like *Procedures for Handling Cytotoxic Drugs*
- Metric-apothecary weight and measure conversion charts

Compounding Sterile Preparations
Effective June 1, 2014, a ASC pharmacy shall not compound sterile preparations unless the pharmacy has applied for and obtained a Class C-S pharmacy

Section Twenty-Two: Class D Clinic Pharmacy

Pharmacist-In-Charge
- Must have one pharmacist-in-charge (PIC) who is employed or under written agreement, at least on a part-time basis, but may be employed on a full-time basis if desired, and who may be PIC of more than one clinic pharmacy
- Written agreement between the clinic and the PIC, and available to the board

Pharmacist-In-Charge Responsibilities
Responsibilities include:
- Continuous supervision of registered nurses, licensed vocational nurses, physician assistants, pharmacy technicians, pharmacy technician trainees, and assistants carrying out the pharmacy related aspects of provision
- Documented periodic on-site visits, either personally or by the consultant pharmacist or staff pharmacist, to insure that the clinic is following set policies and procedures
- Development of a formulary for the clinic, in conjunction with the clinic's pharmacy and therapeutics committee, consisting of drugs and/or devices needed to meet the objectives of the clinic
- Procurement and storage of drugs and/or devices, but he or she may receive input from other appropriate staff of the clinic
- Determining specifications of all drugs and/or devices procured by the clinic

- Maintenance of records of all transactions of the pharmacy as may be required by applicable law and as may be necessary to maintain accurate control over and accountability for all drugs and/or devices
- Development and at least annual review of a policy and procedure manual for the pharmacy in conjunction with the clinic's pharmacy and therapeutics committee
- Meeting inspection and other requirements of the Texas Pharmacy Act and these sections
- Dispensing of prescription orders
- Conducting in-service training at least annually for supportive personnel who provide drugs; such training shall be related to actions, contraindications, adverse reactions, and pharmacology of drugs contained in the formulary

Consultant Pharmacist
- Consultant pharmacist may be the pharmacist-in-charge
- Consultant pharmacist may be retained by more than one clinic

Staff Pharmacists
- PIC must have sufficient number of additional pharmacists as may be required to operate the clinic pharmacy competently, safely, and adequately to meet the needs of the patients of the clinic
- Staff pharmacists and/or the consultant pharmacist shall assist the PIC in meeting the PIC's responsibilities
- Staff pharmacists and/or the consultant pharmacist shall be responsible for any delegated act performed by supportive personnel under his or her supervision

Supportive Personnel

- Supportive personnel shall possess education and training necessary to carry out their responsibilities
- Supportive personnel shall be qualified to perform the pharmacy tasks assigned to them
- Duties may include:
  - Prepackaging and labeling unit of use packages, under the direct supervision of a pharmacist with the pharmacist conducting in-process and final checks and affixing his or her signature to the appropriate quality control records
  - Maintaining inventories of drugs and/or devices and
  - Maintaining pharmacy records
- PIC shall designate from among the supportive personnel a person to supervise the day-to-day pharmacy-related operations of the clinic
- Owner of a Class D pharmacy shall have responsibility for all administrative and operational functions of the pharmacy. The PIC may advise the owner on administrative and operational concerns. The owner shall have responsibility for, at a minimum, the following, and if the owner is not a Texas licensed pharmacist, the owner shall consult with the PIC or another Texas licensed pharmacist:
  - Establishment of policies for procurement of prescription drugs and devices and other products provided or dispensed from the Class D pharmacy
  - Establishment and maintenance of effective controls against the theft or diversion of prescription drugs
  - Providing the pharmacy with the necessary equipment and resources commensurate with its level and type of practice; and

- o Establishment of policies and procedures regarding maintenance, storage, and retrieval of records in a data processing system such that the system is in compliance with state and federal requirements

Registration
- All clinic pharmacies must be registered with the board
- Provide a copy of their policy and procedure manual, which includes the formulary, to the board with the initial license application
- Registration form shall be signed by the PIC of the clinic pharmacy
- Owner or managing officer of the clinic shall sign the registration form and shall agree to comply with the rules adopted by the board governing clinic pharmacies
- Registration form shall be certified and state whether the clinic pharmacy is a sole ownership and give the name of the owner, or if a partnership, name all the managing partners, or if a corporation, name all the managing officers
- When a clinic pharmacy changes ownership, a new and separate license application must be filed with the board and the old license returned to the board's office
- A clinic pharmacy shall notify the board in writing of any change in name or location within 10 days
- A separate license is required for each principal place of business and only one pharmacy license may be issued to a specific location
- A clinic pharmacy shall notify the board in writing within 10 days of a change of the PIC or staff pharmacist or consultant pharmacist
- A clinic pharmacy shall notify the board in writing within 10 days of permanent closing

Registration Requirements for Facilities that Operate at Temporary Clinic Sites

A facility that operates a clinic at one or more temporary locations may be licensed as a Class D (clinic) pharmacy and provide dangerous drugs from these temporary locations provided:

- Clinic pharmacy complies with the registration requirements listed above
- Clinic pharmacy has a permanent location where all dangerous drugs and records are stored
- No dangerous drugs are stored or left for later pickup by the patient at the temporary location(s), and all drugs are returned to the permanent location each day and stored:
  - Within the clinic pharmacy; or
  - Within the pharmacy's mobile unit provided the mobile clinic is parked at the location of the clinic pharmacy in a secure area with adequate measures to prevent unauthorized access, and the drugs are maintained at proper temperatures
- Permanent location is the address of record for the pharmacy
- Facility has no more than six temporary locations in operation simultaneously
- Clinic pharmacy notifies the board of the locations of the temporary locations where drugs will be provided and the schedule for operation of such clinics
- Clinic pharmacy notifies the board within 10 days of a change in address or closing of a temporary location or a change in schedule of operation of a clinic

Environment
- The clinic pharmacy shall have a designated area(s) for the storage of dangerous drugs and/or devices
- No person may operate a pharmacy which is unclean, unsanitary, or under any condition which endangers the health, safety, or welfare of the public
- The pharmacy shall comply with all federal, state, and local health laws and ordinances
- A sink with hot and cold running water shall be available to all pharmacy personnel and shall be maintained in a sanitary condition at all times

Security
- Only authorized personnel may have access to storage areas for dangerous drugs and/or devices
- All storage areas for dangerous drugs and/or devices shall be locked by key, combination, or other mechanical or electronic means, so as to prohibit access by unauthorized individuals
- PIC responsible for the security of all storage areas for dangerous drugs and/or devices including provisions for adequate safeguards against theft or diversion of dangerous drugs and devices, and records for such drugs and devices
- PIC shall consult with clinic personnel with respect to security of the pharmacy, including provisions for adequate safeguards against theft or diversion of dangerous drugs and/or devices, and records for such drugs and/or devices
- Housekeeping and maintenance duties shall be carried out in the pharmacy, while the PIC, consultant pharmacist, staff pharmacist, or supportive personnel is on the premises

Equipment

Each clinic pharmacy shall maintain the following equipment and supplies:

- If the clinic pharmacy prepackages drugs for provision:
    - Typewriter or comparable equipment; and
    - Adequate supply of child-resistant, moisture-proof, and light-proof containers and prescription, poison, and other applicable identification labels used in dispensing and providing of drugs
- If the clinic pharmacy maintains dangerous drugs requiring refrigeration and/or freezing, a refrigerator and/or freezer
- If the clinic pharmacy compounds prescription drug orders, a properly maintained Class A prescription balance (with weights) or equivalent analytical balance. It is the responsibility of the pharmacist-in-charge to have such balance inspected at least every three years by the appropriate authority as prescribed by local, state, or federal law or regulations

Library

A reference library shall be maintained which includes the following in hard copy or electronic format:

- Current copies of the following:
    - Texas Pharmacy Act and rules and
    - Texas Dangerous Drug Act
- Current copies of at least two of the following references:
    - Facts and Comparisons with current supplements
    - AHFS Drug Information
    - United States Pharmacopeia Dispensing Information (USPDI)
    - Physician's Desk Reference (PDR)

- o American Drug Index
- o Reference text on drug interactions, such as Drug Interaction Facts. A separate reference is not required if other references maintained by the pharmacy contain drug interaction information including information needed to determine severity or significance of the interaction and appropriate recommendations or actions to be taken
- o Reference texts in any of the following subjects: toxicology, pharmacology, or drug interactions
- o Reference texts pertinent to the major function(s) of the clinic

Formulary

- Each Class D pharmacy shall have a formulary which lists all drugs and devices that are administered, dispensed, or provided by the Class D pharmacy
- The formulary shall be limited to the following types of drugs and devices, exclusive of injectable drugs for administration in the clinic and nonprescription drugs:
  - o Anti-infective drugs
  - o Musculoskeletal drugs
  - o Vitamins
  - o Obstetrical and gynecological drugs and devices
  - o Topical drugs
  - o Serums, toxoids, and vaccines
- The formulary shall not contain the following drugs or types of drugs:
  - o Nalbuphine (Nubain)
  - o Drugs used to treat erectile dysfunction
  - o Schedule I - V controlled substances

Clinics with Indigent Patients

Clinics with a patient population which consists of at least 80% indigent patients may petition the board to operate with a formulary which includes types of drugs and devices, other than those listed above (no nalbuphine, erectile dysfunction drugs or controlled substances) based upon documented objectives of the clinic, under the following conditions

- Such petition shall contain an affidavit with the notarized signatures of the medical director, the pharmacist-in-charge, and the owner/chief executive officer of the clinic, and include the following documentation:
  - Objectives of the clinic
  - Total number of patients served by the clinic during the previous fiscal year or calendar year
  - Total number of indigent patients served by the clinic during the previous fiscal year or calendar year
  - Percentage of clinic patients who are indigent, based upon the patient population during the previous fiscal year or calendar year
  - Proposed formulary and the need for additional types of drugs based upon objectives of the clinic
  - If the provision of any drugs on the proposed formulary requires special monitoring, the clinic pharmacy shall submit relevant sections of the clinic's policy and procedure manual regarding the provision of drugs that require special monitoring.
- Such petition shall be resubmitted every two years in conjunction with the application for renewal of the pharmacy license.
  - Such renewal petition shall contain the documentation required as listed above

- If at the time of renewal of the pharmacy license, the patient population for the previous fiscal year or calendar year is below 80% indigent patients, the clinic shall be required to submit an application for a Class A pharmacy license or shall limit the clinic formulary to those types of drugs and devices listed in the previous section
- If a clinic pharmacy wishes to add additional drugs to the expanded formulary, the pharmacy shall petition the board in writing prior to adding such drugs to the formulary. The petition shall identify drugs to be added and the need for the additional drugs based upon objectives of the clinic as specified previously
- The following additional requirements shall be satisfied for clinic pharmacies with expanded formularies
  - Supportive personnel who are providing drugs shall be licensed nurses or practitioners
  - The pharmacist-in-charge, consultant pharmacist, or staff pharmacist shall make on-site visits to the clinic at least monthly
  - If the pharmacy provides drugs which require special monitoring (i.e., drugs which require follow-up laboratory work or drugs which should not be discontinued abruptly), the pharmacy shall have policies and procedures for the provision of the prescription drugs to patients and the monitoring of patients who receive such drugs
  - The pharmacist-in-charge, consultant pharmacists, or staff pharmacists shall conduct retrospective drug regimen reviews of a random sample of patients of the clinic on at least a quarterly basis. The pharmacist-in-charge shall be responsible for ensuring that a report regarding the drug regimen review, including the

number of patients reviewed, is submitted to the clinic's medical director and the pharmacy and therapeutics committee of the clinic
- o If a pharmacy provides antipsychotic drugs:
  - ▪ A physician of the clinic shall initiate the therapy
  - ▪ A practitioner shall monitor and order ongoing therapy
  - ▪ The patient shall be physically examined by the physician at least on a yearly basis
- The board may consider the following items in approving or disapproving a petition for an expanded formulary:
  - o Degree of compliance on past compliance inspections
  - o Size of the patient population of the clinic
  - o Number and types of drugs contained in the formulary
  - o Objectives of the clinic

Storage

- Drugs and/or devices which bear the words "Caution, Federal Law Prohibits Dispensing without prescription" or "Rx only" shall be stored in secured storage areas
- All drugs shall be stored at the proper temperatures
- Any drug or device bearing an expiration date may not be provided, dispensed, or administered beyond the expiration date of the drug or device
- Outdated drugs or devices shall be removed from stock and shall be quarantined together until such drugs or devices are disposed
- Controlled substances may not be stored at the clinic pharmacy

Drug Samples

- Drug samples of drugs listed on the clinic pharmacy's formulary and supplied by manufacturers shall be properly stored, labeled, provided, or dispensed by the clinic pharmacy in the same manner as prescribed by these sections for dangerous drugs
- Samples of controlled substances may not be stored, provided, or dispensed in the clinic pharmacy

Prepackaging and Labeling for Provision

- Drugs may be prepackaged and labeled for provision in the clinic pharmacy. Such prepackaging shall be performed by a pharmacist or supportive personnel under the direct supervision of a pharmacist and shall be for the internal use of the clinic
- Drugs must be prepackaged in suitable containers
- The label of the prepackaged unit shall bear:
  - Name, address, and telephone number of the clinic
  - Directions for use, which may include incomplete directions for use provided:
    - Labeling with incomplete directions for use has been authorized by the pharmacy and therapeutics committee
    - Precise requirements for completion of the directions for use are developed by the pharmacy and therapeutics committee and maintained in the pharmacy policy and procedure manual and
    - Directions for use are completed by practitioners, pharmacists, licensed nurses or physician assistants

- o Name and strength of the drug--if generic name, the name of the manufacturer or distributor of the drug
- o Quantity
- o Lot number and expiration date
- o Appropriate ancillary label(s)
- Records of prepackaging shall be maintained according to the Records section

Labeling for Provision of Drugs and/or Devices in an Original Manufacturer's Container

- Drugs and/or devices in an original manufacturer's container shall be labeled prior to provision
- Drugs and/or devices in an original manufacturer's container may be labeled by:
  - o Pharmacist in a pharmacy licensed by the board or
  - o Supportive personnel in a Class D pharmacy, provided the drugs and/or devices and control records are quarantined together until checked and released by a pharmacist
- Keep records of labeling for provision of drugs and/or devices in an original manufacturer's container

Provision

- Drugs and devices may only be provided to patients of the clinic
- At the time of the initial provision, a licensed nurse or practitioner shall provide verbal and written information to the patient or patient's agent on side effects, interactions, and precautions concerning the drug or device provided. If the provision of subsequent drugs is delivered to the patient at the patient's residence or other designated location, the following is applicable:

- o Written information shall be delivered with the medication
- o The pharmacy shall maintain and use adequate storage or shipment containers and use shipping processes to ensure drug stability and potency. Such shipping processes shall include the use of appropriate packaging material and/or devices to ensure that the drug is maintained at an appropriate temperature range to maintain the integrity of the medication throughout the delivery process
- o The pharmacy shall use a delivery system which is designed to ensure that the drugs are delivered to the appropriate patient
- The provision of drugs or devices shall be under the continuous supervision of a pharmacist according to standing delegation orders or standing medical orders and in accordance with written policies and procedures and completion of the label as specified below
- Drugs and/or devices may only be provided in accordance with the system of control and accountability for drugs and/or devices provided by the clinic; such system shall be developed and supervised by the PIC
- Only drugs and/or devices listed in the clinic formulary may be provided
- Drugs and/or devices may only be provided in prepackaged quantities in suitable containers and/or original manufacturer's containers which are appropriately labeled
- Such drugs and/or devices shall be labeled by a pharmacist licensed by the board; however, when drugs and/or devices are provided under the supervision of a physician according to standing delegation orders or standing medical orders, supportive personnel may at

the time of provision print on the label the following
information:
- Patient's name; however, the patient's partner or
  family member is not required to be on the label
  of a drug prescribed for a partner for a sexually
  transmitted disease or for a patient's family
  members if the patient has an illness determined
  by the Centers for Disease Control and
  Prevention, the World Health Organization, or
  the Governor's office to be pandemic
- Any information necessary to complete the
  directions for use
- Date of provision
- Practitioner's name

- Maintain records
- Controlled substances may not be provided or
  dispensed
- Non-sterile and sterile preparations may only be
  provided by the clinic pharmacy in accordance with the
  sections Pharmacies Compounding Non-sterile
  Preparations and Pharmacies Compounding Sterile
  Preparations

Dispensing
Dangerous drugs may only be dispensed by a pharmacist
pursuant to a prescription order

Pharmacy and Therapeutics Committee
- Must have a pharmacy and therapeutics committee
  composed of at least three persons and shall include:
  - PIC
  - Medical director of the clinic, and
  - Person who is responsible for provision of drugs
    and devices
- Develops the policy and procedure manual

- Meets annually to:
  - Review and update the policy and procedure manual; and
  - Review the retrospective drug utilization review reports submitted by the pharmacist-in-charge if the clinic pharmacy has an expanded formulary

Policies and Procedures

- Written policies and procedures shall be developed by the pharmacy and therapeutics committee and implemented by the pharmacist-in-charge
- The policy and procedure manual shall include, but not be limited to, the following:
  - Current list of the names of the pharmacist-in-charge, consultant-pharmacist, staff pharmacist(s), supportive personnel designated to provide drugs or devices, and the supportive personnel designated to supervise the day-to-day pharmacy related operations of the clinic in the absence of the pharmacist
  - Functions of the pharmacist-in-charge, consultant pharmacist, staff pharmacist(s), and supportive personnel
  - Objectives of the clinic
  - Formulary
  - Copy of written agreement between the pharmacist-in-charge and the clinic
  - Date of last review/revision of policy and procedure manual; and
  - Policies and procedures for:
    - Security
    - Equipment
    - Sanitation
    - Licensing
    - Reference materials

- Storage
- Packaging-repackaging
- Dispensing
- Provision
- Retrospective drug regimen review
- Supervision
- Labeling-relabeling
- Samples
- Drug destruction and returns
- Drug and device procuring
- Receiving of drugs and devices
- Delivery of drugs and devices
- Recordkeeping
- Inspection

Supervision

The pharmacist-in-charge, consultant pharmacist, or staff pharmacist shall personally visit the clinic on at least a monthly basis to ensure that the clinic is following established policies and procedures. However, clinics operated by state or local governments and clinics funded by government sources money may petition the board for an alternative visitation schedule under the following conditions:

- Such petition shall contain an affidavit with the notarized signatures of the medical director, the pharmacist-in-charge, and the owner/chief executive officer of the clinic, which states that the clinic has a current policy and procedure manual on file, has adequate security to prevent diversion of dangerous drugs, and is in compliance with all rules governing Class D pharmacies
- The board may consider the following items in determining an alternative schedule:
  - Degree of compliance on past compliance inspections

- o   Size of the patient population of the clinic
- o   Number and types of drugs contained in the formulary
- o   Objectives of the clinic
- Such petition shall be resubmitted every two years in conjunction with the application for renewal of the pharmacy license

General Record Requirements

- Every inventory or other record required to be kept and contained in Clinic Pharmacy (Class D) shall be:
  - o   Kept by the pharmacy and be available, for at least two years from the date of such inventory or record, for inspecting and copying by the board or its representative and to other authorized local, state, or federal law enforcement agencies; and
  - o   Supplied by the pharmacy within 72 hours, if requested by an authorized agent of the Texas State Board of Pharmacy. If the pharmacy maintains the records in an electronic format, the requested records must be provided in a mutually agreeable electronic format if specifically requested by the board or its representative. Failure to provide the records set out in this section, either on site or within 72 hours, constitutes prima facie evidence of failure to keep and maintain records in violation of the Act.
- Records, except when specifically required to be maintained in original or hard-copy form, may be maintained in an alternative data retention system, such as a data processing system or direct imaging system provided:

- Records maintained in the alternative system contain all of the information required on the manual record; and
- Data processing system is capable of producing a hard copy of the record upon the request of the board, its representative, or other authorized local, state, or federal law enforcement or regulatory agencies
- Invoices and records of receipt may be kept at a location other than the pharmacy. Any such records not kept at the pharmacy shall be supplied by the pharmacy within 72 hours, if requested by an authorized agent of the Texas State Board of Pharmacy

On-Site Visits Records

A record of on-site visits by the pharmacist-in-charge, consultant pharmacist, or staff pharmacist shall be maintained and include the following information:
- Date of the visit
- Pharmacist's evaluation of findings
- Signature of the visiting pharmacist

Prepackaging Records

Records of prepackaging shall include the following:
- Name, strength, and dosage form of drug
- Name of the manufacturer
- Manufacturer's lot number
- Expiration date
- Facility's lot number
- Quantity per package and number of packages
- Date packaged
- Name(s), signatures, or electronic signatures of the supportive personnel who prepackages the drug under direct supervision of a pharmacist; and

- Name, signature, or electronic signature of the pharmacist who prepackages the drug or supervises the prepackaging and checks and releases the drug

Labeling Records
Records of labeling of drugs or devices in original manufacturer's containers shall include the following:
- Name and strength of the drug or device labeled
- Name of the manufacturer
- Manufacturer's lot number
- Manufacturer's expiration date
- Quantity per package and number of packages
- Date labeled
- Name of the supportive personnel affixing the label
- Signature of the pharmacist who checks and releases the drug

Provision Records
Records of drugs and/or devices provided shall include logs, patient records, or other acceptable methods for documentation. Documentation shall include:
- Patient name
- Name, signature, or electronic signature of the person who provides the drug or device
- Date provided
- Name of the drug or device and quantity provided

Dispensing Records
Record-keeping requirements for dangerous drugs dispensed by a pharmacist are the same as for a Class A pharmacy

Section Twenty-Three: Class E Non-Resident Pharmacy

Purpose
The purpose of these rules is to provide standards for the operation of non-resident pharmacies (Class E) which dispense a prescription drug or device under a prescription drug order and deliver the drug or device to a patient in this state, by the United States mail, a common carrier, or a delivery service

Personnel
Must be under the continuous on-site supervision of a pharmacist and shall designate one pharmacist licensed to practice pharmacy by the regulatory or licensing agency of the state in which the Class E pharmacy is located to serve as the pharmacist-in-charge of the Class E pharmacy license

Licensing Requirements
- Must be licensed by the board
- On initial application, the pharmacy shall the following:
  - Evidence that the applicant holds a pharmacy license, registration, or permit issued by the state in which the pharmacy is located
  - Name of the owner and pharmacist-in-charge of the pharmacy for service of process
  - Evidence of the applicant's ability to provide to the board a record of a prescription drug order dispensed by the applicant to a resident of this state not later than 72 hours after the time the board requests the record
  - Affidavit by the pharmacist-in-charge which states that the pharmacist has read and

understands the laws and rules relating to a
Class E pharmacy
- o Proof of creditworthiness
- o Inspection report issued not more than two
  years before the date the license application is
  received and conducted by the pharmacy
  licensing board in the state of the pharmacy's
  physical location
    - A Class E pharmacy may submit an
      inspection report issued by an entity
      other than the pharmacy licensing board
      of the state in which the pharmacy is
      physically located if the state's licensing
      board does not conduct inspections as
      follows:
        - An individual approved by the
          board who is not employed by the
          pharmacy but acting as a
          consultant to inspect the pharmacy
        - An agent of the National
          Association of Boards of Pharmacy
        - An agent of another State Board of
          Pharmacy; or
        - An agent of an accrediting body,
          such as the Joint Commission on
          Accreditation of Healthcare
          Organizations
    - The inspection must be substantively
      equivalent to an inspection conducted by
      the board
- On renewal of a license, the pharmacy shall complete
  the renewal application provided by the board and
  provide an inspection report issued not more than three
  years before the date the renewal application is

received and conducted by the pharmacy licensing board in the state of the pharmacy's physical location
- Notify board within 10 days of changes in ownership and must apply for a new and separate license
- Notify board within 10 days of changes in location and/or name and file for an amended license
- Notify board within 10 days of changes in managing officers
- Notify board within 10 days of closing
- Separate license required for each principal place of business and only on pharmacy license may be issued to a specific location
- Don't need to be licensed by the Texas board if an out of state pharmacy restricts its dispensing of prescription drugs or devices to residents of this state to isolated transactions
- Must comply with the provisions specified by the board for centralized dispensing of prescription drug or medication orders, central processing of prescription drugs or medication orders, and compounding of non-sterile preparations
- Prior to August 31, 2014, a Class E pharmacy engaged in the compounding of sterile preparations shall comply with the provisions provided by the board
- Effective August 31, 2014, a Class E pharmacy shall not compound sterile preparations unless the pharmacy has applied for and obtained a Class E-S pharmacy

Prescription Dispensing and Delivery
- All prescription drugs and/or devices shall be dispensed and delivered safely and accurately as prescribed
- The pharmacy shall maintain adequate storage or shipment containers and use shipping processes to ensure drug stability and potency. Such shipping

processes shall include the use of packaging material and devices to ensure that the drug is maintained at an appropriate temperature range to maintain the integrity of the medication throughout the delivery process

- The pharmacy shall utilize a delivery system which is designed to assure that the drugs are delivered to the appropriate patient
- All pharmacists shall exercise sound professional judgment with respect to the accuracy and authenticity of any prescription drug order they dispense. If the pharmacist questions the accuracy or authenticity of a prescription drug order, he/she shall verify the order with the practitioner prior to dispensing
- Prior to dispensing a prescription, pharmacists shall determine, in the exercise of sound professional judgment, that the prescription is a valid prescription. A pharmacist may not dispense a prescription drug if the pharmacist knows or should have known that the prescription was issued on the basis of an Internet-based or telephonic consultation without a valid patient-practitioner relationship this does not prohibit a pharmacist from dispensing a prescription when a valid patient-practitioner relationship is not present in an emergency situation (e.g. a practitioner taking calls for the patient's regular practitioner)

Drug Regimen Review
- For the purpose of promoting therapeutic appropriateness, a pharmacist shall prior to or at the time of dispensing a prescription drug order, review the patient's medication record. Such review shall at a minimum identify clinically significant:
    o Inappropriate drug utilization
    o Therapeutic duplication

- o Drug-disease contraindications
- o Drug-drug interactions
- o Incorrect drug dosage or duration of drug treatment
- o Drug-allergy interactions
- o Clinical abuse/misuse
- Upon identifying any clinically significant conditions or situations the pharmacist shall take appropriate steps to avoid or resolve the problem including consultation with the prescribing practitioner. The pharmacist shall document such occurrences.

Patient Counseling and Provision of Drug Information

- To optimize drug therapy, a pharmacist shall communicate to the patient or the patient's agent, information about the prescription drug or device which in the exercise of the pharmacist's professional judgment the pharmacist deems significant, such as the following:
  - o The name and description of the drug or device
  - o Dosage form, dosage, route of administration, and duration of drug therapy
  - o Special directions and precautions for preparation, administration, and use by the patient
  - o Common severe side or adverse effects or interactions and therapeutic contraindications that may be encountered, including their avoidance, and the action required if they occur
  - o Techniques for self-monitoring of drug therapy;
  - o Proper storage
  - o Refill information
  - o Action to be taken in the event of a missed dose

- Such communication:
  - ○ Shall be provided with each new prescription drug order
  - ○ Shall be provided for any prescription drug order dispensed by the pharmacy on the request of the patient or patient's agent
  - ○ Shall be communicated orally in person unless the patient or patient's agent is not at the pharmacy or a specific communication barrier prohibits such oral communication
  - ○ Shall be reinforced with written information. The following is applicable concerning this written information:
    - ▪ Written information designed for the consumer, such as the USP DI patient information leaflets, shall be provided
    - ▪ When a compounded product is dispensed, information shall be provided for the major active ingredient(s), if available
    - ▪ For new drug entities, if no written information is initially available, the pharmacist is not required to provide information until such information is available, provided:
      - • The pharmacist informs the patient or the patient's agent that the product is a new drug entity and written information is not available
      - • The pharmacist documents the fact that no written information was provided; and
      - • If the prescription is refilled after written information is available,

such information is provided to the patient or patient's agent.

- Effective January 1, 2011, the written information accompanying the prescription or the prescription label shall contain the statement "Do not flush unused medications or pour down a sink or drain." A drug product on a list developed by the Federal Food and Drug Administration of medicines recommended for disposal by flushing is not required to bear this statement.

- Only a pharmacist may orally provide drug information to a patient or patient's agent and answer questions concerning prescription drugs. Non-pharmacist personnel may not ask questions of a patient or patient's agent which are intended to screen and/or limit interaction with the pharmacist

- If prescriptions are routinely delivered outside the area covered by the pharmacy's local telephone service, the pharmacy shall provide a toll-free telephone line which is answered during normal business hours to enable communication between the patient and a pharmacist

- The pharmacist shall place on the prescription container or on a separate sheet delivered with the prescription container in both English and Spanish the local and toll-free telephone number of the pharmacy and the statement: "Written information about this prescription has been provided for you. Please read this information before you take the medication. If you have questions concerning this prescription, a pharmacist is available during normal business hours to answer these questions at (insert the pharmacy's local and toll-free telephone numbers)."

- The provisions of this paragraph do not apply to patients in facilities where drugs are administered to patients by a person required to do so by the laws of the state (i.e., nursing homes)
- Upon delivery of a refill prescription, a pharmacist shall ensure that the patient or patient's agent is offered information about the refilled prescription and that a pharmacist is available to discuss the patient's prescription and provide information
- Nothing in this subparagraph shall be construed as requiring a pharmacist to provide consultation when a patient or patient's agent refuses such consultation. The pharmacist shall document such refusal for consultation

Labeling

At the time of delivery, the dispensing container shall bear a label that contains the following information:

- The name, physical address, and phone number of the pharmacy
- Effective June 1, 2010, if the drug is dispensed in a container other than the manufacturer's original container, the date after which the prescription should not be used or beyond-use-date. Unless otherwise specified by the manufacture, the beyond-use-date shall be one year from the date the drug is dispensed or the manufacturer's expiration date, whichever is earlier. The beyond-use-date may be placed on the prescription label or on a flag label attached to the bottle. A beyond-use-date is not required on the label of a prescription dispensed to a person at the time of release from prison or jail if the prescription is for not more than a 10-day supply of medication
- Effective January 1, 2011, either on the prescription label or the written information accompanying the prescription, the statement, "Do not flush unused

medications or pour down a sink or drain." A drug product on a list developed by the Federal Food and Drug Administration of medicines recommended for disposal by flushing is not required to bear this statement

- Any other information that is required by the pharmacy or drug laws or rules in the state in which the pharmacy is located

Generic Substitution

- Unless compliance would violate the pharmacy or drug laws or rules in the state in which the pharmacy is located a pharmacist in a Class E pharmacy may dispense a generically equivalent drug product
- The pharmacy must include on the prescription order form completed by the patient or the patient's agent information that clearly and conspicuously:
  - States that if a less expensive generically equivalent drug is available for the brand prescribed, the patient or the patient's agent may choose between the generically equivalent drug and the brand prescribed
  - Allows the patient or the patient's agent to indicate the choice of the generically equivalent drug or the brand prescribed

Therapeutic Drug Interchange

A switch to a drug providing a similar therapeutic response to the one prescribed shall not be made without prior approval of the prescribing practitioner. This subsection does not apply to generic substitution.

- The patient shall be notified of the therapeutic drug interchange prior to, or upon delivery, of the dispensed prescription to the patient. Such notification shall include:

- o Description of the change
- o Reason for the change
- o Whom to notify with questions concerning the change; and
- o Instructions for return of the drug if not wanted by the patient
- The pharmacy shall maintain documentation of patient notification of therapeutic drug interchange which shall include:
  - o Date of the notification
  - o Method of notification
  - o Description of the change
  - o Reason for the change

Transfer of Prescription Drug Order Information

Unless compliance would violate the pharmacy or drug laws or rules in the state in which the pharmacy is located, a pharmacist in a Class E pharmacy may not refuse to transfer prescriptions to another pharmacy that is making the transfer request on behalf of the patient

Prescriptions for Schedule II - V Controlled Substances

Unless compliance would violate the pharmacy or drug laws or rules in the state in which the pharmacy is located, a pharmacist in a Class E pharmacy who dispenses a prescription for a Schedule II - V controlled substance issued by a prescriber registered with the Texas Department of Public Safety shall:

- Mail a copy of the prescription to the Texas Department of Public Safety, Texas Prescription Program, P.O. Box 4087, Austin, Texas 78773 within 7 days of dispensing; or
- Electronically send the prescription information to the Texas Department of Public Safety per their

requirements for electronic submissions within 7 days of dispensing

Maintenance of Records

- Every record required to be kept under this section shall be:
    - ○ Kept by the pharmacy and be available, for at least two years from the date of such record, for inspecting and copying by the board or its representative, and other authorized local, state, or federal law enforcement agencies
    - ○ Supplied by the pharmacy within 72 hours, if requested by an authorized agent of the Texas State Board of Pharmacy. If the pharmacy maintains the records in an electronic format, the requested records must be provided in a mutually agreeable electronic format if specifically requested by the board or its representative. Failure to provide the records set out in this section, either on site or within 72 hours, constitutes prima facie evidence of failure to keep and maintain records in violation of the Act
- Records, except when specifically required to be maintained in original or hard-copy form, may be maintained in an alternative data retention system, such as a data processing system or direct imaging system provided:
    - ○ The records maintained in the alternative system contain all of the information required on the manual record; and
    - ○ The data processing system is capable of producing a hard copy of the record upon the request of the board, its representative, or other

authorized local, state, or federal law
enforcement or regulatory agencies

Auto-Refill Programs

A pharmacy may use a program that automatically refills prescriptions that have existing refills available in order to improve patient compliance with and adherence to prescribed medication therapy. The following is applicable in order to enroll patients into an auto-refill program.

- Notice of the availability of an auto-refill program shall be given to the patient or patient's agent, and the patient or patient's agent must affirmatively indicate that they wish to enroll in such a program and the pharmacy shall document such indication
- The patients or patient's agent shall have the option to withdraw from such a program at any time
- Auto-refill programs may be used for refills of dangerous drugs, and schedule IV and V controlled substances. Schedule II and III controlled substances may not be dispensed by an auto-refill program
- As is required for all prescriptions, a drug regimen review shall be completed on all prescriptions filled as a result of the auto-refill program. Special attention shall be noted for drug regimen review warnings of duplication of therapy and all such conflicts shall be resolved with the prescribing practitioner prior to refilling the prescription

Civil Litigation and Complaint Records

A Class E pharmacy shall keep a permanent record of:

- Any civil litigation commenced against the pharmacy by a Texas resident
- Complaints that arise out of a prescription for a Texas resident lost during delivery

Pharmacies Compounding Sterile Preparations (Class E-S)

A non-resident pharmacy engaged in the compounding of sterile preparations shall be licensed as a Class E-S pharmacy

- A Class E-S pharmacy shall register with the board on a pharmacy license application provided by the board
- A Class E-S license may not be issued unless the pharmacy has been inspected by the board or its designee. A Class E-S pharmacy shall reimburse the board for all expenses, including travel, related to the inspection of the Class E-S pharmacy
- On initial application, the pharmacy shall follow the procedures specified previously in this section:
  - Evidence that the applicant holds a pharmacy license, registration, or permit issued by the state in which the pharmacy is located
  - Name of the owner and pharmacist-in-charge of the pharmacy for service of process
  - Evidence of the applicant's ability to provide to the board a record of a prescription drug order dispensed by the applicant to a resident of this state not later than 72 hours after the time the board requests the record
  - Affidavit by the pharmacist-in-charge which states that the pharmacist has read and understands the laws and rules relating to a Class E pharmacy
  - Proof of creditworthiness
- A Class E-S pharmacy may not renew a pharmacy license unless the pharmacy has been inspected by the board or its designee within the last two years
- Notify board within ten days of the change of ownership and apply for a new and separate license
- Notify the board within ten days of changes in location and/or name and file for an amended license

- Notify board within 10 days of change in managing officers
- Notify board within 10 days of closing
- A separate license is required for each principal place of business and only one pharmacy license may be issued to a specific location
- The board may grant an exemption from the licensing requirements of this Act on the application of a pharmacy located in a state of the United States other than this state that restricts its dispensing of prescription drugs or devices to residents of this state to isolated transactions

Section Twenty-Four: Pharmacies Located in a Freestanding Emergency Medical Care Center – Class F

Purpose

The purpose of this section is to provide standards in the conduct, practice activities, and operation of a pharmacy located in a freestanding emergency medical care center (FEMCC) that is licensed by the Texas Department of State Health Services or in a FEMCC operated by a hospital that is exempt from registration as provided by §254.052, Health and Safety Code. Class F pharmacies located in a FEMCC shall comply with this section.

Pharmacist-In-Charge

- Each freestanding emergency medical care center shall have one pharmacist-in-charge (PIC) who is employed or under contract, at least on a consulting or part-time basis, but may be employed on a full-time basis
- Minimum responsibilities include:
    - Establishment of specifications for procurement and storage of all materials, including drugs, chemicals, and biologicals
    - Participation in the development of a formulary for the FEMCC, subject to approval of the appropriate committee of the FEMCC
    - Distribution of drugs to be administered to patients pursuant to an original or direct copy of the practitioner's medication order
    - Filling and labeling all containers from which drugs are to be distributed or dispensed

- Maintaining and making available a sufficient inventory of antidotes and other emergency drugs, both in the pharmacy and patient care areas, as well as current antidote information, telephone numbers of regional poison control center and other emergency assistance organizations, and such other materials and information as may be deemed necessary by the appropriate committee of the FEMCC
- Records of all transactions of the FEMCC pharmacy as may be required by applicable state and federal law, and as may be necessary to maintain accurate control over and accountability for all pharmaceutical materials
- Participation in those aspects of the FEMCC's patient care evaluation program which relate to pharmaceutical material utilization and effectiveness
- Participation in teaching and/or research programs in the FEMCC
- Implementation of the policies and decisions of the appropriate committee(s) relating to pharmaceutical services of the FEMCC
- Effective and efficient messenger and delivery service to connect the FEMCC pharmacy with appropriate areas of the FEMCC on a regular basis throughout the normal workday of the FEMCC
- Labeling, storage, and distribution of investigational new drugs, including maintenance of information in the pharmacy and nursing station where such drugs are being administered, concerning the dosage form, route of administration, strength, actions, uses, side effects, adverse effects, interactions, and

symptoms of toxicity of investigational new drugs

- o Meeting all inspection and other requirements of the Texas Pharmacy Act and this section
- o Maintenance of records in a data processing system such that the data processing system is in compliance with the requirements for a FEMCC

Consultant Pharmacist

- The consultant pharmacist may be the PIC
- A written contract shall exist between the FEMCC and any consultant pharmacist, and a copy of the written contract shall be made available to the board upon request

Pharmacists

- PIC shall be assisted by a sufficient number of additional licensed pharmacists as may be required to operate the FEMCC pharmacy competently, safely, and adequately to meet the needs of the patients of the facility
- All pharmacists shall assist the pharmacist-in-charge in meeting the responsibilities as listed above and in ordering, administering, and accounting for pharmaceutical materials
- All pharmacists shall be responsible for any delegated act performed by pharmacy technicians or pharmacy technician trainees under his or her supervision
- All pharmacists while on duty shall be responsible for complying with all state and federal laws or rules governing the practice of pharmacy
- Duties of the pharmacist-in-charge and all other pharmacists shall include, but need not be limited to, the following:
    - o Receiving and interpreting prescription drug orders and oral medication orders and reducing

these orders to writing either manually or electronically
  - ○ Selection of prescription drugs and/or devices and/or suppliers; and
  - ○ Interpreting patient profiles
- All pharmacists engaged in compounding non-sterile preparations shall meet the training requirements relating to Pharmacies Compounding Non-Sterile Preparations
- All pharmacists engaged in compounding sterile preparations shall meet the training requirements relating to Pharmacies Compounding Sterile Preparations

Pharmacy Technicians and Pharmacy Technician Trainees

- All pharmacy technicians and pharmacy technician trainees shall meet the training requirements relating to Pharmacy Technician and Pharmacy Technician Trainee Training
- Duties may include, but need not be limited to, the following functions, under the direct supervision of a pharmacist:
  - ○ Prepacking and labeling unit and multiple dose packages, provided a pharmacist supervises and conducts a final check and affixes his or her name, initials, electronic signature to the appropriate quality control records prior to distribution
  - ○ Preparing, packaging, compounding, or labeling prescription drugs pursuant to medication orders, provided a pharmacist supervises and checks the preparation
  - ○ Compounding non-sterile preparations pursuant to medication orders provided the pharmacy

technicians or pharmacy technician trainees have completed the training

- Compounding sterile preparations pursuant to mediation orders provided the pharmacy technicians or pharmacy technician trainees:
  - Have completed the required training
  - Supervised by a pharmacist who has completed the sterile preparations training, conducts in-process and final checks and affixes his or her name, initials, or electronic signature to the label or if batch prepared to the appropriate quality control records (the name, initials or electronic signature are not required on the label if it is maintained in a permanent record of the pharmacy)
- Bulk compounding, provided a pharmacist supervises and conducts in-process and final checks and affixes his or her name, initials, or electronic signature to the label or if batch prepared to the appropriate quality control records (the name, initials or electronic signature are not required on the label if it is maintained in a permanent record of the pharmacy)
- Distributing routine orders for stock supplies to patient care areas
- Entering medication order and drug distribution information into a data processing system, provided judgmental decisions are not required and a pharmacist checks the accuracy of the information entered into the system prior to releasing the order or in compliance with the absence of pharmacist requirements
- Maintaining inventories of drug supplies

- o Maintaining pharmacy records
- o Loading bulk unlabeled drugs into an automated drug dispensing system provided a pharmacist supervises, verifies that the system was properly loaded prior to use, and affixes his or her name, initials, or electronic signature to the appropriate quality control records
- Pharmacy technicians and pharmacy technician trainees shall handle medication orders in accordance with standard written procedures and guidelines
- Pharmacy technicians and pharmacy technician trainees shall handle prescription drug orders in the same manner as pharmacy technicians or pharmacy technician trainees working in a Class A pharmacy
- Must be trained in compounding non-sterile and sterile preparations

Owner

The owner of a FEMCC pharmacy shall have responsibility for all administrative and operational functions of the pharmacy. The PIC may advise the owner on administrative and operational concerns. The owner shall have responsibility for, at a minimum, the following, and if the owner is not a Texas licensed pharmacist, the owner shall consult with the PIC or another Texas licensed pharmacist:

- Establishment of policies for procurement of prescription drugs and devices and other products dispensed from the FEMCC pharmacy
- Establishment and maintenance of effective controls against the theft or diversion of prescription drugs
- If the pharmacy uses an automated pharmacy dispensing system, reviewing and approving all policies and procedures for system operation, safety, security, accuracy and access, patient confidentiality, prevention of unauthorized access, and malfunction

- Providing the pharmacy with the necessary equipment and resources commensurate with its level and type of practice and
- Establishment of policies and procedures regarding maintenance, storage, and retrieval of records in a data processing system such that the system is in compliance with state and federal requirements.

Identification of Pharmacy Personnel

All pharmacy personnel will wear an identification tag or badge that displays the person's name and title such as: pharmacy technician, certified pharmacy technician, pharmacy technician trainee, pharmacist intern or pharmacist

Licensing Requirements

- Register annually or biennially with the board
- If the FEMCC pharmacy is owned or operated by a pharmacy management or consulting firm, the following conditions apply:
  - The pharmacy license application shall list the pharmacy management or consulting firm as the owner or operator.
  - The pharmacy management or consulting firm shall obtain DEA and DPS controlled substances registrations that are issued in the name of the firm, unless the following occur:
    - Pharmacy management or consulting firm and the facility cosign a contractual pharmacy service agreement which assigns overall responsibility for controlled substances to the facility and
    - Such pharmacy management or consulting firm maintains dual responsibility for the controlled substances

- Notify board within 10 days of change of ownership for a new and separate license
- Notify board within 10 days of change in location and/or name for an amended license
- Notify board within 10 days of change in managing officers
- Notify board within 10 day of closing
- Separate license required for each principal place of business and only one pharmacy license can be issued to a specific location

Environment
Each freestanding emergency medical care center shall have a designated work area separate from patient areas, and which shall have space adequate for the size and scope of pharmaceutical services and shall have adequate space and security for the storage of drugs.
- Must have locked storage for Schedule II controlled substances and other controlled drugs requiring additional security
- Must have a designated area for the storage of poisons and externals separate from drug storage areas
- Only authorized personnel may have access to storage areas for prescription drugs and/or devices
- All storage areas for prescription drugs and/or devices shall be locked by key, combination or other mechanical or electronic means, so as to prohibit unauthorized access

Library
A reference library shall be maintained that includes the following in hard-copy or electronic format and pharmacy personnel shall be capable of accessing at all times:
- Current copies of the following:
  - Texas Pharmacy Act and rules

- o Texas Dangerous Drug Act and rules
- o Texas Controlled Substances Act and rules
- o Federal Controlled Substances Act and rules or official publication describing the requirements of the Federal Controlled Substances Act and rules;
- At least one current or updated reference from each of the following categories:
  - o Drug interactions. A reference text on drug interactions, such as Drug Interaction Facts. A separate reference is not required if other references maintained by the pharmacy contain drug interaction information including information needed to determine severity or significance of the interaction and appropriate recommendations or actions to be taken
  - o General information. A general information reference text, such as:
    - Facts and Comparisons with current supplements
    - United States Pharmacopeia Dispensing Information Volume I (Drug Information for the Healthcare Provider)
    - AHFS Drug Information with current supplements
    - Remington's Pharmaceutical Sciences; or
    - Clinical Pharmacology
- A current or updated reference on injectable drug products, such as Handbook of Injectable Drugs
- Basic antidote information and the telephone number of the nearest regional poison control center
- If the pharmacy compounds sterile preparations, specialty references appropriate for the scope of services provided by the pharmacy, e.g., if the pharmacy prepares cytotoxic drugs, a reference text on the

preparation of cytotoxic drugs, such as Procedures for Handling Cytotoxic Drugs
- Metric-apothecary weight and measure conversion charts

Procurement, Preparation, and Storage of Drugs
- PIC shall have the responsibility for the procurement and storage of drugs, but may receive input from other appropriate staff of the facility, relative to such responsibility
- PIC shall have the responsibility for determining specifications of all drugs procured by the facility
- FEMCC pharmacies may not sell, purchase, trade, or possess prescription drug samples, unless the pharmacy meets the requirements as specified in §291.16
- All drugs shall be stored at the proper temperatures
- Any drug bearing an expiration date may not be dispensed or distributed beyond the expiration date of the drug
- Outdated drugs shall be removed from dispensing stock and shall be quarantined together until such drugs are disposed of

Formulary
- A formulary may be developed by an appropriate committee of the freestanding emergency medical center
- PIC or consultant pharmacist shall be a full voting member of any committee which involves pharmaceutical services

Prepackaging of Drugs
- Drugs may be prepackaged in quantities suitable for internal distribution only by a pharmacist or by

pharmacy technicians or pharmacy technician trainees under the direction and direct supervision of a pharmacist
- The label of a prepackaged unit shall indicate:
    o Brand name and strength of the drug; or if no brand name, then the generic name, strength, and name of the manufacturer or distributor;
    o Facility's lot number
    o Expiration date
    o Quantity of the drug, if quantity is greater than one
- Records of prepackaging shall be maintained to show:
    o Name of the drug, strength, and dosage form;
    o Facility's lot number
    o Manufacturer or distributor
    o Manufacturer's lot number
    o Expiration date
    o Quantity per prepackaged unit
    o Number of prepackaged units
    o Date packaged
    o Name, initials, or electronic signature of the prepacker
    o Signature or electronic signature of the responsible pharmacist
- Stock packages, repackaged units, and control records shall be quarantined together until checked/released by the pharmacist

Loading Bulk Unlabeled Drugs into Automated Drug Dispensing Systems
- Automated drug dispensing systems may be loaded with bulk unlabeled drugs only by a pharmacist or by pharmacy technicians or pharmacy technician trainees under the direction and direct supervision of a pharmacist

- The label of an automated drug dispensing system container shall indicate the brand name and strength of the drug; or if no brand name, then the generic name, strength, and name of the manufacturer or distributor
- Records of loading bulk unlabeled drugs into an automated drug dispensing system shall be maintained to show:
  - Name of the drug, strength, and dosage form
  - Manufacturer or distributor
  - Manufacturer's lot number
  - Expiration date
  - Date of loading
  - Name, initials, or electronic signature of the person loading the automated drug dispensing system
  - Signature or electronic signature of the responsible pharmacist
- The automated drug dispensing system shall not be used until a pharmacist verifies that the system is properly loaded and affixes his or her signature or electronic signature to the record

Medication Orders

- Drugs may be administered to patients in FEMCCs only on the order of a practitioner. No change in the order for drugs may be made without the approval of a practitioner
- Drugs may be distributed only pursuant to the original or a direct copy of the practitioner's medication order
- Pharmacy technicians and pharmacy technician trainees may not receive oral medication orders
- FEMCC pharmacies shall be exempt from the labeling provisions and patient notification requirements of §562.006 and §562.009 of the Act, as respects drugs distributed pursuant to medication orders

- In FEMCCs with a full-time pharmacist, if a practitioner orders a drug for administration to a bona fide patient of the facility when the pharmacy is closed, the following is applicable
  - Prescription drugs and devices only in sufficient quantities for immediate therapeutic needs of a patient may be removed from the FEMCC pharmacy
  - Only a designated licensed nurse or practitioner may remove such drugs and devices
  - A record shall be made at the time of withdrawal by the authorized person removing the drugs and devices. The record shall contain the following information:
    - Name of the patient
    - Name of device or drug, strength, and dosage form
    - Dose prescribed
    - Quantity taken
    - Time and date
    - Signature or electronic signature of person making withdrawal
  - The original or direct copy of the medication order may substitute for such record, provided it contains the information listed above
  - The pharmacist shall verify the withdrawal as soon as practical, but in no event more than 72 hours from the time of such withdrawal
- In FEMCCs with a part-time or consultant pharmacist, if a practitioner orders a drug for administration to a bona fide patient of the FEMCC when the pharmacist is not on duty, or when the pharmacy is closed, the following is applicable.

- Prescription drugs and devices only in sufficient quantities for therapeutic needs may be removed from the FEMCC pharmacy
- Only a designated licensed nurse or practitioner may remove such drugs and devices
- A record shall be made at the time of withdrawal by the authorized person removing the drugs and devices; the record shall meet the same requirements as specified previously
- The pharmacist shall verify each distribution after a reasonable interval, but in no event may such interval exceed seven days

Floor Stock

In facilities using a floor stock method of drug distribution, the following is applicable for removing drugs or devices in the absence of a pharmacist

- Prescription drugs and devices may be removed from the pharmacy only in the original manufacturer's container or prepackaged container
- Only a designated licensed nurse or practitioner may remove such drugs and devices
- A record shall be made at the time of withdrawal by the authorized person removing the drug or device; the record shall contain the following information:
  - Name of the drug, strength, and dosage form
  - Quantity removed
  - Location of floor stock
  - Date and time; and
  - Signature or electronic signature of person making the withdrawal
- A pharmacist shall verify the withdrawal according to the following schedule
  - In facilities with a full-time pharmacist, the withdrawal shall be verified as soon as practical,

but in no event more than 72 hours from the
time of such withdrawal
- o In facilities with a part-time or consultant
  pharmacist, the withdrawal shall be verified
  after a reasonable interval, but in no event may
  such interval exceed seven days

Policies and Procedures

Written policies and procedures for a drug distribution system,
appropriate for the freestanding emergency medical center,
shall be developed and implemented by the pharmacist-in-
charge with the advice of the appropriate committee. The
written policies and procedures for the drug distribution
system shall include, but not be limited to, procedures
regarding the following:

- Controlled substances
- Investigational drugs
- Prepackaging and manufacturing
- Medication errors
- Orders of physician or other practitioner
- Floor stocks
- Adverse drug reactions
- Drugs brought into the facility by the patient
- Self-administration
- Emergency drug tray
- Formulary, if applicable
- Drug storage areas
- Drug samples
- Drug product defect reports
- Drug recalls
- Outdated drugs
- Preparation and distribution of IV admixtures
- Procedures for supplying drugs for postoperative use, if
  applicable

- Use of automated drug dispensing systems
- Use of data processing systems

Drugs Supplied for Outpatient Use

- Drugs may only be supplied to patients who have been admitted to the freestanding emergency medical center
- Drugs may only be supplied in accordance with the system of control and accountability established for drugs supplied from the freestanding emergency medical center; such system shall be developed and supervised by the pharmacist-in-charge or staff pharmacist designated by the pharmacist-in-charge
- Only drugs listed on the approved outpatient drug list may be supplied; such list shall be developed by the PIC and the medical staff and shall consist of drugs of the nature and type to meet the immediate postoperative needs of the freestanding emergency medical center patient
- Drugs may only be supplied in prepackaged quantities not to exceed a 72-hour supply in suitable containers and appropriately prelabeled (including necessary auxiliary labels) by the pharmacy, provided, however that topicals and ophthalmics in original manufacturer's containers may be supplied in a quantity exceeding a 72-hour supply
- At the time of delivery of the drug, the practitioner shall complete the label, such that the prescription container bears a label with at least the following information:
  - Date supplied
  - Name of practitioner
  - Name of patient
  - Directions for use
  - Brand name and strength of the drug; or if no brand name, then the generic name of the drug

dispensed, strength, and the name of the manufacturer or distributor of the drug; and
  - Unique identification number
- After the drug has been labeled by the practitioner, the practitioner or a licensed nurse under the supervision of the practitioner shall give the appropriately labeled, prepackaged medication to the patient
- A perpetual record of drugs which are supplied from the FEMCC shall be maintained which includes:
  - Name, address, and phone number of the facility
  - Date supplied
  - Name of practitioner
  - Name of patient
  - Directions for use
  - Brand name and strength of the drug; or if no brand name, then the generic name of the drug dispensed, strength, and the name of the manufacturer or distributor of the drug; and
  - Unique identification number
- The pharmacist-in-charge, or a pharmacist designated by the pharmacist-in-charge, shall review the records at least once every seven days

Maintenance of Records

- Every inventory or other record required to be kept under the provisions of this section (relating to Freestanding Emergency Medical Care Center) shall be:
  - Kept by the pharmacy and be available, for at least two years from the date of such inventory or record, for inspecting and copying by the board or its representative, and other authorized local, state, or federal law enforcement agencies; and
  - Supplied by the pharmacy within 72 hours, if requested by an authorized agent of the Texas

State Board of Pharmacy. If the pharmacy maintains the records in an electronic format, the requested records must be provided in a mutually agreeable electronic format if specifically requested by the board or its representative. Failure to provide the records set out in this subsection, either on site or within 72 hours, constitutes prima facie evidence of failure to keep and maintain records in violation of the Act.

- Records of controlled substances listed in Schedules I and II shall be maintained separately from all other records of the pharmacy.
- Records of controlled substances listed in Schedules III - V shall be maintained separately or readily retrievable from all other records of the pharmacy. For purposes of this subsection, readily retrievable means that the controlled substances shall be asterisked, red-lined, or in some other manner readily identifiable apart from all other items appearing on the record.
- Records, except when specifically required to be maintained in original or hard-copy form, may be maintained in an alternative data retention system, such as a data processing or direct imaging system, e.g., microfilm or microfiche, provided:
  - Records in the alternative data retention system contain all of the information required on the manual record; and
  - Alternative data retention system is capable of producing a hard copy of the record upon the request of the board, its representative, or other authorized local, state, or federal law enforcement or regulatory agencies

Outpatient Records

- Only a registered pharmacist may receive, certify, and receive prescription drug orders
- Outpatient records shall be maintained the same as required by Community Pharmacy (Class A)
- Outpatient prescriptions, including, but not limited to, discharge prescriptions, that are written by the practitioner, must be written on a form which meets the requirements of the Act, §562.006. Medication order forms or copies thereof do not meet the requirements for outpatient forms
- Controlled substances listed in Schedule II must be written on an official prescription form in accordance with the Texas Controlled Substances Act, §481.075, and rules promulgated pursuant to the Texas Controlled Substances Act, unless exempted by the Texas Controlled Substances Rules, 37 TAC §13.74. Outpatient prescriptions for Schedule II controlled substances that are exempted from the official prescription requirement must be manually signed by the practitioner

Patient Records

- Each original medication order or set of orders issued together shall bear the following information:
  - Patient name
  - Drug name, strength, and dosage form
  - Directions for use
  - Date
  - Signature or electronic signature of the practitioner or that of his or her authorized agent, defined as a licensed nurse employee or consultant/full or part-time pharmacist of the FEMCC

- Original medication orders shall be maintained with the medication administration record in the medical records of the patient
- Controlled substances records shall be maintained as follows:
  - All records for controlled substances shall be maintained in a readily retrievable manner
  - Controlled substances records shall be maintained in a manner to establish receipt and distribution of all controlled substances
- Records of controlled substances listed in Schedule II shall be maintained as follows:
  - Records of controlled substances listed in Schedule II shall be maintained separately from records of controlled substances in Schedules III, IV, and V, and all other records
  - A FEMCC pharmacy shall maintain a perpetual inventory of any controlled substance listed in Schedule II
  - Distribution records for Schedule II - V controlled substances floor stock shall include the following information:
    - Patient's name
    - Practitioner who ordered drug
    - Name of drug, dosage form, and strength
    - Time and date of administration to patient and quantity administered
    - Signature or electronic signature of individual administering controlled substance
    - Returns to the pharmacy
    - Waste (waste is required to be witnessed and cosigned, manually or electronically, by another individual)
- Floor stock records shall be maintained as follows

- Distribution records for Schedules III - V controlled substances floor stock shall include the following information:
  - Patient's name
  - Practitioner who ordered controlled substance
  - Name of controlled substance, dosage form, and strength
  - Time and date of administration to patient
  - Quantity administered
  - Signature or electronic signature of individual administering drug
  - Returns to the pharmacy
  - Waste (waste is required to be witnessed and cosigned, manually or electronically, by another individual)
  - The record required by this clause shall be maintained separately from patient records
  - A pharmacist shall review distribution records with medication orders on a periodic basis to verify proper usage of drugs, not to exceed 30 days between such reviews
- General requirements for records maintained in a data processing system are as follows
  - If an FEMCC pharmacy's data processing system is not in compliance with the board's requirements, the pharmacy must maintain a manual recordkeeping system
  - Requirements for backup systems. The facility shall maintain a backup copy of information stored in the data processing system using disk, tape, or other electronic backup system and update this backup copy on a regular basis to assure that data is not lost due to system failure

- o Change or discontinuance of a data processing system
  - Records of distribution and return for all controlled substances and nalbuphine (Nubain). A pharmacy that changes or discontinues use of a data processing system must:
    - Transfer the records to the new data processing system; or
    - Purge the records to a printout which contains the same information as required on the audit trail printout. The information on this printout shall be sorted and printed by drug name and list all distributions/returns chronologically
  - Other records. A pharmacy that changes or discontinues use of a data processing system must:
    - Transfer the records to the new data processing system; or
    - Purge the records to a printout which contains all of the information required on the original document
  - Maintenance of purged records. Information purged from a data processing system must be maintained by the pharmacy for two years from the date of initial entry into the data processing system.

- Data processing system maintenance of records for the distribution and return of all controlled substances and nalbuphine (Nubain) to the pharmacy
  - Each time a controlled substance, or nalbuphine (Nubain) is distributed from or returned to the pharmacy, a record of such distribution or return shall be entered into the data processing system
  - The data processing system shall have the capacity to produce a hard-copy printout of an audit trail of drug distribution and return for any strength and dosage form of a drug (by either brand or generic name or both) during a specified time period. This printout shall contain the following information:
    - Patient's name and room number or patient's facility identification number
    - Prescribing or attending practitioner's name
    - Name, strength, and dosage form of the drug product actually distributed
    - Total quantity distributed from and returned to the pharmacy
    - If not immediately retrievable via electronic image, the following shall also be included on the printout:
      - Prescribing or attending practitioner's address
      - Practitioner's DEA registration number, if the medication order is for a controlled substance
  - An audit trail printout for each strength and dosage form of these drugs distributed during the preceding month shall be produced at least monthly and shall be maintained in a separate file at the facility. The information on this

printout shall be sorted by drug name and list all distributions/returns for that drug chronologically

- o The pharmacy may elect not to produce the monthly audit trail printout if the data processing system has a workable (electronic) data retention system which can produce an audit trail of drug distribution and returns for the preceding two years. The audit trail required in this clause shall be supplied by the pharmacy within 72 hours, if requested by an authorized agent of the Texas State Board of Pharmacy, or other authorized local, state, or federal law enforcement or regulatory agencies.
- Failure to maintain records. Failure to provide records set out in this subsection, either on site or within 72 hours for whatever reason, constitutes prima facie evidence of failure to keep and maintain records
- Data processing system downtime. In the event that an FEMCC pharmacy which uses a data processing system experiences system downtime, the pharmacy must have an auxiliary procedure which will ensure that all data is retained for on-line data entry as soon as the system is available for use again

Distribution of Controlled Substances to Another Registrant

A pharmacy may distribute controlled substances to a practitioner, another pharmacy, or other registrant, without being registered to distribute, under the following conditions

- The registrant to whom the controlled substance is to be distributed is registered under the Controlled Substances Act to dispense that controlled substance
- The total number of dosage units of controlled substances distributed by a pharmacy may not exceed

226

5.0% of all controlled substances dispensed by the pharmacy during the 12-month period in which the pharmacy is registered; if at any time it does exceed 5.0%, the pharmacy is required to obtain an additional registration to distribute controlled substances
- If the distribution is for a Schedule III, IV, or V controlled substance, a record shall be maintained which indicates:
    o The actual date of distribution
    o The name, strength, and quantity of controlled substances distributed
    o The name, address, and DEA registration number of the distributing pharmacy
    o The name, address, and DEA registration number of the pharmacy, practitioner, or other registrant to whom the controlled substances are distributed
- If the distribution is for a Schedule I or II controlled substance, the following is applicable
    o The pharmacy, practitioner, or other registrant who is receiving the controlled substances shall issue Copy 1 and Copy 2 of a DEA order form (DEA 222C) to the distributing pharmacy
    o The distributing pharmacy shall:
        ▪ Complete the area on the DEA order form (DEA 222C) titled "To Be Filled in by Supplier"
        ▪ Maintain Copy 1 of the DEA order form (DEA 222C) at the pharmacy for two years; and
        ▪ Forward Copy 2 of the DEA order form (DEA 222C) to the divisional office of the Drug Enforcement Administration

Other Records

Other records to be maintained by the pharmacy include:

- A permanent log of the initials or identification codes which will identify each pharmacist by name. The initials or identification code shall be unique to ensure that each pharmacist can be identified, i.e., identical initials or identification codes cannot be used
- Copy 3 of DEA order form (DEA 222C), which has been properly dated, initialed, and filed, and all copies of each unaccepted or defective order form and any attached statements or other documents
- A hard copy of the power of attorney to sign DEA 222C order forms (if applicable)
- Suppliers' invoices of dangerous drugs and controlled substances; a pharmacist shall verify that the controlled drugs listed on the invoices were actually received by clearly recording his/her initials and the actual date of receipt of the controlled substances
- Supplier's credit memos for controlled substances and dangerous drugs
- A hard copy of inventories required by §291.17 of this title (relating to Inventory Requirements) except that a perpetual inventory of controlled substances listed in Schedule II may be kept in a data processing system if the data processing system is capable of producing a hard copy of the perpetual inventory on-site
- Hard-copy reports of surrender or destruction of controlled substances and/or dangerous drugs to an appropriate state or federal agency
- A hard-copy Schedule V nonprescription register book
- Records of distribution of controlled substances and/or dangerous drugs to other pharmacies, practitioners, or registrants; and

- A hard copy of any notification required by the Texas Pharmacy Act or these rules, including, but not limited to, the following:
    o Reports of theft or significant loss of controlled substances to DEA, DPS, and the board
    o Notification of a change in pharmacist-in-charge of a pharmacy
    o Reports of a fire or other disaster which may affect the strength, purity, or labeling of drugs, medications, devices, or other materials used in the diagnosis or treatment of injury, illness, and disease

Permission to Maintain Central Records

Any pharmacy that uses a centralized recordkeeping system for invoices and financial data shall comply with the following procedures.

- Controlled substance records. Invoices and financial data for controlled substances may be maintained at a central location provided the following conditions are met
    o Prior to the initiation of central recordkeeping, the pharmacy submits written notification by registered or certified mail to the divisional director of the Drug Enforcement Administration, and submits a copy of this written notification to the Texas State Board of Pharmacy. Unless the registrant is informed by the divisional director of the Drug Enforcement Administration that permission to keep central records is denied, the pharmacy may maintain central records commencing 14 days after receipt of notification by the divisional director
    o The pharmacy maintains a copy of the notification required in this subparagraph

- The records to be maintained at the central record location shall not include executed DEA order forms, prescription drug orders, or controlled substance inventories, which shall be maintained at the pharmacy
- Invoices and financial data for dangerous drugs may be maintained at a central location
- Must have access to records if on microfilm, computer media, or in any form requiring special equipment to render the records easily readable
- Must deliver records to the pharmacy location within two business days of written request of a board agent or any other authorized official

Section Twenty-Five: Central Prescription Drug or Medication Order Processing Pharmacy – Class G

Purpose
Any facility established for the primary purpose of processing prescription drug or medication drug orders shall be licensed as a Class G pharmacy under the Act. A Class G pharmacy shall not store bulk drugs, or dispense a prescription drug order. Nothing in this subsection shall prohibit an individual pharmacist employee who is licensed in Texas from remotely accessing the pharmacy's electronic data base from a location other than a licensed pharmacy in order to process prescription or medication drug orders, provided the pharmacy establishes controls to protect the privacy and security of confidential records, and the Texas-licensed pharmacist does not engage in the receiving of written prescription or medication orders or the maintenance of prescription or medication drug orders at the non-licensed remote location.

Centralized Prescription Drug or Medication Order Processing
The processing of a prescription drug or medication orders by a Class G pharmacy on behalf of another pharmacy, a health care provider, or a payor. Centralized prescription drug or medication order processing does not include the dispensing of a prescription drug but includes any of the following:
- Receiving, interpreting, or clarifying prescription drug or medication drug orders
- Data entering and transferring of prescription drug or medication order information

- Performing drug regimen review
- Obtaining refill and substitution authorizations
- Verifying accurate prescription data entry
- Interpreting clinical data for prior authorization for dispensing
- Performing therapeutic interventions
- Providing drug information concerning a patient's prescription

Full-Time Pharmacist
A pharmacist who works in a pharmacy from 30 to 40 hours per week or, if the pharmacy is open less than 60 hours per week, one-half of the time the pharmacy is open

Pharmacist-In-Charge
- Each Class G pharmacy shall have one pharmacist-in-charge (PIC) who is employed on a full-time basis, who may be the PIC for only one such pharmacy
- PIC shall have responsibility for the practice of pharmacy at the pharmacy for which he or she is the PIC and may advise the owner on administrative or operational concerns. The PIC shall have responsibility for, at a minimum, the following:
    o Education and training of pharmacy technicians and pharmacy technician trainees
    o Maintaining records of all transactions of the Class G pharmacy required by applicable state and federal laws and sections
    o Adherence to policies and procedures regarding the maintenance of records in a data processing system such that the data processing system is in compliance with Class G pharmacy requirements
    o Legal operation of the pharmacy, including meeting all inspection and other requirements of

all state and federal laws or sections governing the practice of pharmacy

Owner

The owner of a Class G pharmacy shall have responsibility for all administrative and operational functions of the pharmacy. The PIC may advise the owner on administrative and operational concerns. The owner shall have responsibility for, at a minimum, the following, and if the owner is not a Texas licensed pharmacist, the owner shall consult with the pharmacist-in-charge or another Texas licensed pharmacist:

- Providing the pharmacy with the necessary equipment and resources commensurate with its level and type of practice
- Establishment of policies and procedures regarding maintenance, storage, and retrieval of records in a data processing system such that the system is in compliance with state and federal requirements

Pharmacists

- The pharmacist-in-charge shall be assisted by sufficient number of additional licensed pharmacists as may be required to operate the Class G pharmacy competently, safely, and adequately to meet the needs of the patients of the pharmacy
- All pharmacists shall assist the pharmacist-in-charge in meeting his or her responsibilities
- Pharmacists are solely responsible for the direct supervision of pharmacy technicians and pharmacy technician trainees and for designating and delegating duties to pharmacy technicians and pharmacy technician trainees. Each pharmacist shall be responsible for any delegated act performed by pharmacy technicians and pharmacy technician trainees under his or her supervision

233

- Pharmacists shall directly supervise pharmacy technicians and pharmacy technician trainees who are entering prescription data into the pharmacy's data processing system by one of the following methods.
    - Physically present supervision. A pharmacist shall be physically present to directly supervise a pharmacy technician or pharmacy technician trainee who is entering prescription order or medication order data into the data processing system. Each prescription or medication order entered into the data processing system shall be verified at the time of data entry
    - Electronic supervision. A pharmacist may electronically supervise a pharmacy technician or pharmacy technician trainee who is entering prescription order or medication order data into the data processing system provided the pharmacist:
        - Is on-site, in the pharmacy where the technician/trainee is located
        - Has immediate access to any original document containing prescription or medication order information or other information related to the dispensing of the prescription or medication order. Such access may be through imaging technology provided the pharmacist has the ability to review the original, hardcopy documents if needed for clarification; and
        - Verifies the accuracy of the data entered information prior to the release of the information to the system for storage
    - Electronic verification of data entry by pharmacy technicians or pharmacy technician trainees. A

pharmacist may electronically verify the data entry of prescription information into a data processing system provided:

- A pharmacist is on-site in the pharmacy where the pharmacy technicians/trainees are located
- The pharmacist electronically conducting the verification is either a:
  - Texas licensed pharmacist; or
  - Pharmacist employed by a Class E pharmacy that has the same owner as the Class G pharmacy where the pharmacy technicians/trainees are located or that has entered into a written contract or agreement with the Class G pharmacy, which outlines the services to be provided and the responsibilities and accountabilities of each pharmacy in compliance with federal and state laws and regulations
- The pharmacy establishes controls to protect the privacy and security of confidential records
- The pharmacy keeps permanent records of prescriptions electronically verified for a period of two years

Duties

Duties which may only be performed by a pharmacist are as follows:

- Receiving oral prescription drug or medication orders and reducing these orders to writing, either manually or electronically

- Interpreting prescription drug or medication orders
- Selecting drug products
- Verifying the data entry of the prescription drug or medication order information at the time of data entry prior to the release of the information to a Class A, Class C, or Class E pharmacy for dispensing
- Communicating to the patient or patient's agent information about the prescription drug or device which in the exercise of the pharmacist's professional judgment, the pharmacist deems significant
- Communicating to the patient or the patient's agent on his or her request information concerning any prescription drugs dispensed to the patient by the pharmacy
- Assuring that a reasonable effort is made to obtain, record, and maintain patient medication records
- Interpreting patient medication records and performing drug regimen reviews; and
- Performing a specific act of drug therapy management for a patient delegated to a pharmacist by a written protocol from a physician licensed in this state in compliance with the Medical Practice Act

Pharmacy Technicians and Pharmacy Technician Trainees

- All pharmacy technicians and pharmacy technician trainees shall meet the training requirements specified
- Duties include:
  - Pharmacy technicians and pharmacy technician trainees may not perform any of the duties listed in the pharmacist section
  - A pharmacist may delegate to pharmacy technicians and pharmacy technician trainees any nonjudgmental technical duty associated

with the preparation and distribution of prescription drugs provided:
- Pharmacist verifies the accuracy of all acts, tasks, and functions
- Under direct supervision of and responsible to a pharmacist
  - o May perform only nonjudgmental technical duties associated with the preparation of prescription drugs, as follows:
    - Initiating and receiving refill authorization requests
    - Entering prescription or medication order data into a data processing system
- A Class G pharmacy may have a ratio of on-site pharmacists to pharmacy technicians and pharmacy technician trainees of 1:8 provided:
  - o At least seven are pharmacy technicians and not pharmacy technician trainees
  - o The pharmacy has written policies and procedures regarding the supervision of pharmacy technicians and pharmacy technician trainees

Identification of Pharmacy Personnel

All pharmacy personnel will wear an identification tag or badge that displays the person's name and title such as: pharmacy technician, certified pharmacy technician, pharmacy technician trainee, pharmacist intern or pharmacist

Operational Standards

- A Class A, Class C, or Class E Pharmacy may outsource prescription drug or medication order processing to a Class G pharmacy provided the pharmacies:
  - o Have:
    - The same owner; or

- Entered into a written contract or agreement which outlines the services to be provided and the responsibilities and accountabilities of each pharmacy in compliance with federal and state laws and regulations and
  - Share a common electronic file or have appropriate technology to allow access to sufficient information necessary or required to perform a non-dispensing function

Licensing Requirements

- A Class G pharmacy shall register with the board on a pharmacy license application provided by the board
- Notify board within 10 days of change in ownership to apply for a new and separate license
- Notify board within 10 days of changes in location and/or name to file for an amended license
- Notify board within 10 days of changes in managing officers
- Notify board within 10 day of closing
- A separate license is required for each principal place of business and only one pharmacy license may be issued to a specific location

Environment

- The pharmacy shall be arranged in an orderly fashion and kept clean. All required equipment shall be in good operating condition
- The pharmacy shall be properly lighted and ventilated
- Each pharmacist while on duty shall be responsible for the security of the prescription department, including provisions for effective control against theft or diversion of prescription drug records

- Pharmacies shall employ appropriate measures to ensure that security of prescription drug records is maintained at all times to prohibit unauthorized access

Policy and Procedures

A policy and procedure manual shall be maintained by the Class G pharmacy and be available for inspection. The manual shall:

- Outline the responsibilities of each of the pharmacies
- Include a list of the name, address, telephone numbers, and all license/registration numbers of the pharmacies involved in centralized prescription drug or medication order processing; and
- Include policies and procedures for:
  - o Protecting the confidentiality and integrity of patient information
  - o Maintenance of appropriate records to identify the name(s), initials, or identification code(s) and specific activity(ies) of each pharmacist or pharmacy technician who performed any processing
  - o Complying with federal and state laws and regulations
  - o Operating a continuous quality improvement program for pharmacy services designed to objectively and systematically monitor and evaluate the quality and appropriateness of patient care, pursue opportunities to improve patient care, and resolve identified problems; and
  - o Annually reviewing the written policies and procedures and documenting such review

Records

- Every record required to be kept under the provisions this section shall be:
  - Kept by the pharmacy and be available, for at least two years from the date of such inventory or record, for inspecting and copying by the board or its representative and to other authorized local, state, or federal law enforcement agencies; and
  - Supplied by the pharmacy within 72 hours, if requested by an authorized agent of the Texas State Board of Pharmacy. If the pharmacy maintains the records in an electronic format, the requested records must be provided in a mutually agreeable electronic format if specifically requested by the board or its representative. Failure to provide the records set out in this section, either on site or within 72 hours, constitutes prima facie evidence of failure to keep and maintain records in violation of the Act
- The pharmacy shall maintain appropriate records which identify, by prescription drug or medication order, the name(s), initials, or identification code(s) of each pharmacist, pharmacy technician, or pharmacy technician trainee who performs a processing function for a prescription drug or medication order. Such records may be maintained:
  - Separately by each pharmacy and pharmacist; or
  - In a common electronic file as long as the records are maintained in such a manner that the data processing system can produce a printout which lists the functions performed by each pharmacy and pharmacist

- In addition, the pharmacy shall comply with the record keeping requirements applicable to the class of pharmacy to the extent applicable for the specific processing activity and this section

Section Twenty-Six: Limited Prescription Delivery Pharmacy – Class H

Purpose
- The purpose of this section is to provide standards for a limited prescription delivery pharmacy
- Any facility established for the primary purpose of limited prescription delivery by a Class A pharmacy shall be licensed as a Class H pharmacy
- A Class H pharmacy shall not store bulk drugs, or dispense a prescription drug order
- A Class H pharmacy may deliver prescription drug orders for dangerous drugs
- A Class H pharmacy may not deliver prescription drug orders for controlled substances

Pharmacist-In-Charge
- Each Class H pharmacy shall have one pharmacist-in-charge (PIC) who is employed or under written agreement, at least on a part-time basis, but may be employed on a full-time basis, and who may be the PIC for more than one limited prescription delivery pharmacy
- PIC responsible for the practice of pharmacy and may advise owner on administrative or operational concerns
- Responsibilities include:
  - Education and training of pharmacy technicians and pharmacy technician trainees

- o Maintaining records of all transactions of the Class H pharmacy required by applicable state and federal laws and sections
- o Adherence to policies and procedures regarding the maintenance of records
- o Legal operation of the pharmacy, including meeting all inspection and other requirements of all state and federal laws or sections governing the practice of pharmacy

Owner

The owner of a Class H pharmacy shall have responsibility for all administrative and operational functions of the pharmacy. The PIC may advise the owner on administrative and operational concerns. The owner shall have responsibility for, at a minimum, the following, and if the owner is not a Texas licensed pharmacist, the owner shall consult with the PIC or another Texas licensed pharmacist:

- Providing the pharmacy with the necessary equipment and resources commensurate with its level and type of practice; and
- Establishment of policies and procedures regarding maintenance, storage, and retrieval of records in compliance with state and federal requirements

Pharmacists

- The PIC shall be assisted by sufficient number of additional licensed pharmacists as may be required to operate the Class H pharmacy competently, safely, and adequately to meet the needs of the patients of the pharmacy
- All pharmacists shall assist the PIC in meeting his or her responsibilities

- Pharmacists shall be responsible for any delegated act performed by the pharmacy technicians under his or her supervision

Pharmacy Technicians and Pharmacy Technician Trainees

- All pharmacy technicians and pharmacy technician trainees shall meet the training requirements
- Duties include:
  - Delivery of previously verified prescription drug orders to a patient or patient's agent provided a record of prescriptions delivered is maintained; and
  - Maintaining pharmacy records

Identification of Pharmacy Personnel

All pharmacy personnel will wear an identification tag or badge that displays the person's name and title such as: pharmacy technician, certified pharmacy technician, pharmacy technician trainee, pharmacist intern or pharmacist

General Requirements

A Class A or Class E Pharmacy may outsource limited prescription delivery to a Class H pharmacy provided the pharmacies have entered into a written contract or agreement which outlines the services to be provided and the responsibilities and accountabilities of each pharmacy in compliance with federal and state laws and regulations

Licensing Requirements

- Must register with the board for a license
- A Class H pharmacy must be owned by a hospital district and located in a county without another pharmacy

- Notify board within 10 days of change of ownership and apply for a new and separate license
- Notify board within 10 days of changes location and/or name and file for an amended license
- Notify board within 10 days of closing
- A separate license is required for each principal place of business and only one pharmacy license may be issued to a specific location

Environment
- The pharmacy shall have a designated area for the storage of previously verified prescription drug orders
- The pharmacy shall be arranged in an orderly fashion and kept clean
- A sink with hot and cold running water shall be available to all pharmacy personnel and shall be maintained in a sanitary condition at all times

Security
- Only authorized personnel may have access to storage areas for dangerous drugs
- When a pharmacist, pharmacy technician or pharmacy technician trainee is not present all storage areas for dangerous drugs devices shall be locked by key, combination, or other mechanical or electronic means, so as to prohibit access by unauthorized individuals
- The pharmacist-in-charge shall be responsible for the security of all storage areas for dangerous drugs including provisions for adequate safeguards against theft or diversion of dangerous drugs, and records for such drugs
- Housekeeping and maintenance duties shall be carried out in the pharmacy, while the pharmacist-in-charge,

consultant pharmacist, staff pharmacist, or pharmacy technician/trainee is on the premises

Library
A reference library shall be maintained which includes current copies of the following in hard copy or electronic format:
- Texas Pharmacy Act and rules
- Texas Dangerous Drug Act
- At least one current or updated patient information reference such as:
  - United States Pharmacopeia Dispensing Information, Volume II (Advice to the Patient); or
  - A reference text or information leaflets which provide patient information; and
- Basic antidote information and the telephone number of the nearest Regional Poison Control Center

Delivery of Drugs
- The pharmacist-in-charge, consultant pharmacist, staff pharmacist, pharmacy technician, or pharmacy technician trainee must be present at the pharmacy to deliver prescriptions
- Prescriptions for controlled substances may not be stored or delivered by the pharmacy
- Prescriptions may be stored at the pharmacy for no more than 15 days. If prescriptions are not picked up by the patient, the medications are to be destroyed utilizing a reverse distribution service
- PIC, consultant pharmacist, or staff pharmacist shall personally visit the pharmacy on at least a weekly basis and conduct monthly audits of prescriptions received and delivered by the pharmacy

Records

- Every record required to be kept under the provisions this section shall be:
  - Kept by the pharmacy and be available, for at least two years from the date of such inventory or record, for inspecting and copying by the board or its representative and to other authorized local, state, or federal law enforcement agencies; and
  - Supplied by the pharmacy within 72 hours, if requested by an authorized agent of the Texas State Board of Pharmacy. If the pharmacy maintains the records in an electronic format, the requested records must be provided in a mutually agreeable electronic format if specifically requested by the board or its representative. Failure to provide the records set out in this section, either on site or within 72 hours, constitutes prima facie evidence of failure to keep and maintain records in violation of the Act
- A record of on-site visits by the PIC, consultant pharmacist, or staff pharmacist shall be maintained and include the following information:
  - Date of the visit
  - Pharmacist's evaluation of findings
  - Signature of the visiting pharmacist
- Records of prescription drug orders delivered to the Class H pharmacy shall include:
  - Patient name
  - Name and quantity of drug delivered
  - Name of pharmacy and address delivering the prescription drug order
  - Date received at the Class H pharmacy
- Records of drugs delivered to a patient or patient's agent shall include:

- Patient name
  - Name, signature, or electronic signature of the person who picks up the prescription drug
  - Date delivered
  - Name of the drug and quantity delivered
- For the purposes of these sections, a pharmacy licensed under the Act is the only entity which may legally own and maintain prescription drug records

Section Twenty-Seven: Services Provided by Pharmacies

Remote Pharmacy Services

Provide standards for the provision of pharmacy services by a Class A or Class C pharmacy in a facility that is not at the same location as the Class A or Class C pharmacy through an automated pharmacy system

- Automated pharmacy system – A mechanical system that dispenses prescription drugs and maintains related transaction information
- Remote site – A facility not located at the same location as a Class A or Class C pharmacy, at which remote pharmacy services are provided using an automated pharmacy dispensing system
- Provider pharmacy – The community pharmacy (Class A) or the institutional pharmacy (Class C) providing remote pharmacy services.
- Remote pharmacy service – The provision of pharmacy services, including the storage and dispensing of prescription drugs, in remote sites

General Requirements

- A provider pharmacy may provide remote pharmacy services using an automated pharmacy system to a jail or prison operated by or for the State of Texas, a jail or prison operated by local government, or a healthcare facility regulated under Chapter 142, 242, 247, or 252 *Health and Safety Code*, provided drugs are

administered by a licensed healthcare professional working in the jail, prison, or healthcare facility
- Inpatients of the remote site only
- May provide remote services to more than one site
- Automated pharmacy system must be tested for accuracy prior to being used
- If provider pharmacy is Class C, then must comply with Class A rules
- A pharmacist from the provider pharmacy shall be accessible at all times to respond to patients' or other health professionals' questions and needs pertaining to drugs dispensed through the use of the automated pharmacy system. Such access may be through a 24-hour pager service or telephone that is answered 24 hours a day

Operational Standards
- Class A or Class C pharmacy must apply to the board to provide remote pharmacy services
- Resubmit application every 2 years in conjunction with provider pharmacy's license renewal
- Approval certificate must be displayed at the remote site
- Notify board in writing within 10 days of a change of location, discontinuance of service, or closure of
  - Remote site where an automated pharmacy system is operated by the pharmacy; **or**
  - Remote pharmacy service at a remote site

Environment/Security of Automated Pharmacy System

- Must be locked by key, combination, or other mechanical or electronic means to prohibit access by unauthorized personnel
- Must be under continuous supervision of a provider pharmacy pharmacist.
    - Supervision may be electronic instead of physically on-site

Prescription Dispensing and Delivery

- Only can dispense drugs upon a prescription drug order
- Pharmacist controls the release of the initial dose
- Additional approved doses may be released after initial approval
- Drug regimen review required
- Drugs shall be packaged in the original manufacturer's container or be prepackaged in the provider pharmacy and labeled in compliance with the board's prepackaging requirements for the class of pharmacy
- Drugs dispensed from the automated pharmacy system may be returned to the pharmacy for reuse provided the drugs are in sealed, tamper-evident packaging that has not been opened

Stocking an Automated Pharmacy System

- Completed by a pharmacist, pharmacy technician, or pharmacy technician trainee under the direct supervision of a pharmacist, **or**
- If removable cartridges or containers to hold drugs are used, the prepackaging of the cartridges or containers shall occur at the provider pharmacy, unless provided

by an FDA-approved repackager. The prepackaged cartridges or containers may be sent to the remote site to be loaded into the machine by personnel designated by the pharmacist-in-charge, provided:

- Pharmacist verifies the cartridge or container has been properly filled and labeled
- Individual cartridges or containers are transported to the remote site in a secure, tamper-evident container
- Automated pharmacy system uses bar coding, microchip, or other technologies to ensure that the containers are accurately loaded in the automated pharmacy system
- All drugs to be stocked in the automated pharmacy system shall be delivered to the remote site by the provider pharmacy

Quality Assurance Program

- Required continuous supervision of the automated pharmacy system
- Test accuracy at a minimum of every 6 months or whenever an upgrade or change is made to the system

Records

- Provider pharmacy shall maintain original prescription drug orders for drugs dispensed from an automated pharmacy system
- The automated pharmacy system shall electronically record all transactions involving drugs stored in, removed, or dispensed from the system

Inventory

A provider pharmacy shall:

- Keep a record of all drugs sent to and returned from a remote site separate from the records of the provider pharmacy and from any other remote site's records
- Keep a perpetual inventory of controlled substances and other drugs required to be inventoried that are received and dispensed or distributed from each remote site
- Inventory of each remote site and the provider pharmacy shall be taken on the same day
- Inventory records shall be included with, but listed separately from, the drugs of other remote sites and separately from the drugs of the provider pharmacy

Emergency Medication Kits

Class A or Class C pharmacy in a facility that is not at the same location as the Class A or Class C pharmacy through an emergency medication kit

Definitions

- Emergency medication kits – controlled substances and dangerous drugs maintained by a provider pharmacy to meet the emergency medication needs of a resident
    - At an institution licensed under Chapter 242 or 252, Health and Safety Code; or
    - At an institution licensed under Chapter 242, Health and Safety Code, and that is a veterans' home as defined by the §164.002, Natural Resources Code, if the provider pharmacy is a United States Department of Veterans Affairs

pharmacy or another federally operated pharmacy

- Prepackaging – the act of repackaging and relabeling quantities of drug products from a manufacturer's original commercial container, or quantities of unit dosed drugs, into another cartridge or container for dispensing by a pharmacist using an emergency medication kit
- Provider pharmacy – the community pharmacy (Class A), the institutional pharmacy (Class C), the non-resident (Class E) pharmacy located not more than 20 miles from an institution licensed under Chapter 242 or 252, Health and Safety Code, or the United States Department of Veterans Affairs pharmacy or another federally operated pharmacy providing remote pharmacy services
- Remote pharmacy service – the provision of pharmacy services, including the storage and dispensing of prescription drugs, in remote sites
- Remote site – a facility not located at the same location as a Class A, Class C, Class E pharmacy or a United States Department of Affairs pharmacy or another federally operated pharmacy, at which remote pharmacy services are provided using an emergency medication kit

General Requirements

- A provider pharmacy may provide remote pharmacy services using an emergency medication kit to an institution regulated under Chapter 242, or 252, Health and Safety Code
- May provide remote pharmacy services at more than one remote site

- A provider pharmacy shall not place an emergency medication kit in a remote site which already has a kit from another provider pharmacy, unless
  - The provider pharmacies enter into a written agreement as to the emergency medications supplied by each pharmacy. The provider pharmacies shall not duplicate drugs stored in the emergency medication kits. The written agreement shall include reasons why an additional pharmacy is required to meet the emergency medication needs of the residents of the institution
- The pharmacist-in-charge of the provider pharmacy is responsible for all pharmacy operations involving the emergency medication kit located at the remote site including supervision of the emergency medication kit and compliance with this section

Operational Standards

- Class A, Class C, or Class E Pharmacy – must apply to the board to provide remote pharmacy services using an emergency medication kit
- Reapply every 2 years with provider pharmacy's license renewal
- Display approval certificate at the remote site

Notification Requirements

A provider pharmacy shall notify the board in writing within ten (10) days of a change of location, discontinuance of service, or closure of

- A remote site where an emergency medication kit is operated by the pharmacy; **or**
- A remote pharmacy service at a remote site

Environment/Security

- Emergency medication kits shall have adequate security and procedures to
    - Prohibit unauthorized access
    - Comply with federal and state laws and regulations
    - Maintain patient confidentiality
- Access shall be limited to pharmacists and licensed healthcare personnel employed by the facility

Prescription Drugs and Delivery

- Drugs may only be accessed pursuant to an order from a practitioner
- Prescription drug order for drugs used from the emergency medication kit shall be forwarded to the provider pharmacy
- Remote site shall notify the provider pharmacy of each entry into an emergency medication kit

Drugs

- May consist of dangerous drugs and controlled substances
- Limited to drugs necessary to meet residents' emergency medication needs (a drug that cannot be supplied by a pharmacy within a reasonable time period)
- Consultant pharmacist, pharmacist-in-charge of the provider pharmacy, medical director, and the director of nurses will decide which drugs
- Current list of the drugs stored in each remote site's emergency medication kit shall be maintained by the

provider pharmacy and a copy kept with the emergency medication kit
- Automated pharmacy system may be used as an emergency medication kit provided the system limits emergency access to only those drugs approved for the emergency medication kit
- Drugs shall be packaged in the original manufacturer's container or prepackaged in the provider pharmacy and labeled in compliance with the board's prepackaging requirements for the class of pharmacy

Stocking Emergency Medication Kits

- Completed at the provider pharmacy or remote site by a pharmacist, pharmacy technician, or pharmacy technician trainee under the direct supervision of a pharmacist
- If the emergency medication kit is an automated pharmacy system that uses removable cartridges or containers to hold drugs, the prepackaging of the cartridges or containers shall occur at the provider pharmacy, unless provided by an FDA-approved repackager
- The prepackaged cartridges or containers may be sent to the remote site to be loaded into the machine by personnel designated by the pharmacist-in-charge, provided
  - o Pharmacist verifies the cartridge or container has been properly filled and labeled
  - o Individual cartridges or containers are transported to the remote site in a secure, tamper-evident container; **and**
  - o Automated pharmacy system uses bar coding, microchip, or other technologies to ensure that

the containers are accurately loaded in the automated pharmacy system

Inventory

- Keep a record of all drugs sent to and returned from a remote site separate from the records of the provider pharmacy and from any other remote site's records
- Keep a perpetual inventory of controlled substances and other drugs required to be inventoried that are received and dispensed or distributed from each remote site
- Provider pharmacy shall conduct an inventory at each remote site
    - Inventory of each remote site and the provider pharmacy shall be taken on the same day
    - Inventory of each remote site shall be included with, but listed separately from, the drugs of other remote sites and separately from the drugs of the provider pharmacy

Telepharmacy

The purpose of this section is to provide standards for the provision of pharmacy services by a Class A or Class C pharmacy in a healthcare facility that is not at the same location as a Class A or Class C pharmacy through a telepharmacy system

Definitions

- Provider pharmacy – the community pharmacy (Class A) or the institutional pharmacy (Class C) providing remote pharmacy services

- Remote site – a facility not located at the same location as a Class A or Class C pharmacy, at which remote pharmacy services are provided, using a telepharmacy dispensing system
- Remote pharmacy service – the provision of pharmacy services, including the storage and dispensing of prescription drugs, drug regimen review, and patient counseling, at a remote site
- Still image capture – a specific image captured electronically from a video or other image capture device
- Store and forward – a video or still image record which is saved electronically for future review
- Telepharmacy system – a system that monitors the dispensing of prescription drugs and provides for related drug use review and patient counseling services by an electronic method which shall include the use of the following types of technology:
  - Audio and video
  - Still image capture
  - Store and forward
- Unit-of-use – a sufficient quantity of a drug for one normal course of therapy as determined by the pharmacist-in-charge and the prescribing practitioner(s) at the healthcare facility

General Requirements

- A provider pharmacy may provide remote pharmacy services using a telepharmacy system to
  - A rural health clinic regulated under 42 U.S.C. Section 1395x(aa)
  - A health center as defined by 42 U.S.C. Section 254b; **or**

- - a healthcare facility located in a medically underserved area as defined by state or federal law
- A provider pharmacy may not provide remote pharmacy services if a Class A or Class C pharmacy that dispenses prescription drug orders to outpatients is located in the same community. For the purposes of this subsection, a community is defined as:
  - The census tract in which the remote site is located, if the remote site is located in a Metropolitan Statistical Area (MSA) as defined by the United States Census Bureau in the most recent U.S. Census; **or**
  - Within 10 miles of the remote site, if the remote site is not located in a MSA
- Each pharmacist at the provider pharmacy may supervise no more than three (3) remote sites that are simultaneously open to provide services
- Must test the telepharmacy system for accuracy prior to use

Operational Standards

- Class A or Class C pharmacy must apply to the board to provide remote pharmacy services using a telepharmacy system
- Reapply every two (2) years in conjunction with provider pharmacy's license renewal
- Registration certificate must be displayed at the remote site

Notification Requirements

A provider pharmacy shall notify the board in writing within ten (10) days of a change of location, discontinuance of service, or closure of

- Remote site where a telepharmacy system is operated by the pharmacy; **or**
- Remote pharmacy service at a remote site

Environment/Security

- Must be continuous supervision of a provider pharmacy pharmacist at all times the site is open to provide pharmacy services. To qualify as continuous supervision, the pharmacist is not required to be physically present at the remote site and may supervise electronically through the use of the following types of technology:
    - Audio and video
    - Still image capture; **and**
    - Store and forward
- Drugs for use in the telepharmacy system shall be stored in an area that is
    - Separate from any other drugs used by the healthcare facility; **and**
    - Locked by key, combination or other mechanical or electronic means, to prohibit access by unauthorized personnel
- Access to the area where drugs are stored at the remote site and operation of the telepharmacy system shall be limited to pharmacists employed by the provider pharmacy or personnel who
    - Are licensed pharmacy technicians or pharmacy technician trainees

- o Are designated in writing by the pharmacist-in-charge; **and**
- o Have completed documented training concerning their duties associated with the telepharmacy pharmacy system
- Drugs may only be delivered to the remote site by the provider pharmacy and shall be
  - o Shipped in a sealed container with a list of drugs delivered
  - o Signed for on receipt by an employee of the healthcare facility
  - o Quarantined in a locked area, if personnel designated to receive the drugs by the pharmacist-in-charge is not available; **and**
  - o Checked by personnel designated by the pharmacist-in-charge to verify that drugs sent by the provider pharmacy were actually received. The designated person who checks the order shall document the verification by signing and dating the list of drugs delivered

Prescription Dispensing and Delivery

- Drugs may only be dispensed upon an original prescription drug order
- Drugs may only be dispensed in unit-of-use containers that are
  - o Prepackaged in suitable containers at the provider pharmacy and appropriately labeled; **or**
  - o In original manufacturer's containers
- The following duties shall be performed only by a pharmacist at the provider pharmacy:
  - o Receiving an oral prescription drug order
  - o Interpreting a prescription drug order

- Verifying the accuracy of prescription data entry
- Selecting the drug product
- Interpreting the patient's medication record
- Conducting a drug regimen review
- Authorizing the telepharmacy system to print a prescription label at the remote site
- Performing the final check of the dispensed prescription
- Counseling the patient
- A pharmacist at the provider pharmacy shall conduct a drug regimen review prior to delivery of the dispensed prescription to the patient or patient's agent
- The dispensed prescription shall be properly labeled at the remote site **but**
  - The label shall contain the name, address, and phone number of the provider pharmacy and the name and address of the remote site; **and**
  - The unique identification number of the prescription on the label shall in some manner identify the remote site which dispensed the prescription using a telepharmacy system
- A pharmacist at the provider pharmacy shall perform the final check of the dispensed prescription before delivery to the patient – visual check using electronic methods
- A pharmacist at the provider pharmacy shall counsel the patient or patient's agent - may be performed using electronic methods
- Non-pharmacist personnel may not ask questions of a patient or patient's agent which are intended to screen or limit interaction with the pharmacist
- If the remote site has direct access to the provider pharmacy's data processing system, only a pharmacist, pharmacy technician, or pharmacy technician trainee may enter prescription information into the data

processing system. The original prescription shall be sent to the provider pharmacy, and a pharmacist shall verify the accuracy of the data entry
- Drugs which require reconstitution through the addition of a specified amount of water may be dispensed by the remote site only if a pharmacy technician, pharmacy technician trainee, or licensed healthcare provider reconstitutes the product

Quality Assurance Program

A pharmacist must
- Continuously supervise of the telepharmacy system at all times the site is open to provide pharmacy services
- Test the operation of the telepharmacy system at least every 6 months and whenever any upgrade or change is made to system

Inventory

- Keep a record of all drugs sent to and returned from a remote site separate from the records of the provider pharmacy and from any other remote site's records
- Keep a perpetual inventory of controlled substances and other drugs required to be inventoried that are received and dispensed or distributed from each remote site
- Provider pharmacy shall conduct an inventory at each remote site
    o Inventory of each remote site and the provider pharmacy shall be taken on the same day
    o Inventory of each remote site shall be included with, but listed separately from, the drugs of other remote sites and separately from the drugs of the provider pharmacy

Central Prescription Drug or Medication Order Processing

The purpose of this section is to provide standards for centralized prescription drug or medication order processing by a Class A (Community), Class C (Institutional), or Class E (Non-Resident) pharmacy.

Definition

The processing of a prescription drug or medication orders by a Class A, Class C, or Class E pharmacy on behalf of another pharmacy, a health care provider, or a payor. Centralized prescription drug or medication order processing does not include the dispensing of a prescription drug order but does include any of the following:

- receiving, interpreting, or clarifying prescription drug or medication drug orders
- Data entering and transferring of prescription drug or medication order information
- Performing drug regimen review
- Obtaining refill and substitution authorizations
- Interpreting clinical data for prior authorization for dispensing
- Performing therapeutic interventions
- Providing drug information concerning a patient's prescription

Operational Standards

Class A, Class C, or Class E harmacy may outsource prescription drug or medication order processing to another Class A, Class C, or Class E pharmacy provided the pharmacies have

- The same owner; **or**

- Entered into a written contract or agreement which outlines the services to be provided and the responsibilities and accountabilities of each pharmacy in compliance with federal and state laws and regulations and share a common electronic file or have appropriate technology to allow access to sufficient information necessary or required to process a non-dispensing function

A pharmacy that performs centralized prescription drug or medication order processing shall comply with the provisions applicable to their class of pharmacy including
- Duties which must be performed by a pharmacist; **and**
- Supervision requirements for pharmacy technicians and pharmacy technician trainees

Notifications to Patients

A pharmacy that outsources prescription drug or medication order processing to another pharmacy shall, prior to outsourcing their prescription
- Notify patients that prescription processing may be outsourced to another pharmacy; **and**
- Give the name of that pharmacy
  - If the pharmacy is part of a network of pharmacies under common ownership and any of the network pharmacies may process the prescription, the patient shall be notified of this fact. Such notification may be provided through a one-time written notice to the patient or through use of a sign in the pharmacy

Records

All pharmacies shall maintain appropriate records which identify, by prescription drug or medication order, the name(s), initials, or identification code(s) of each pharmacist, pharmacy technician, or pharmacy technician trainee who performs a processing function for a prescription drug or medication order. Such records may be maintained

- Separately by each pharmacy and pharmacist; **or**
- In a common electronic file as long as the records are maintained in such a manner that the data processing system can produce a printout which lists the functions performed by each pharmacy and pharmacist

Centralized Prescription Dispensing

The purpose of this section is to provide standards for centralized prescription dispensing by a Class A, Class C pharmacy, or Class E pharmacy.

Definition

The dispensing or refilling of a prescription drug order by a Class A, Class C, or Class E pharmacy at the request of another Class A or Class C, and at the return of the dispensed prescriptions to the requesting pharmacy for delivery to the patient or patient's agent or, at the request of the requesting pharmacy, direct delivery to the patient

Operational Standards

Class A or Class C pharmacy may outsource prescription drug order dispensing to another Class A, Class C, or Class E pharmacy provided the pharmacies

- Have the same owner or entered into a written contract or agreement which outlines the services to be provided and the responsibilities and accountabilities of each pharmacy in compliance with federal and state laws and regulations; **and**
- Share a common electronic file or have appropriate technology to allow access to sufficient information necessary or required to dispense or process a prescription drug order

The pharmacist-in-charge of the dispensing pharmacy shall ensure that

- Adequate storage or shipment containers and shipping processes to ensure drug stability and potency – keep in the correct temperature range
- Dispensed prescriptions are shipped in containers which are sealed in a manner as to show evidence of opening or tampering

Notifications to Patients

A pharmacy that outsources prescription dispensing to another pharmacy shall, prior to outsourcing the prescription,

- Notify patients that their prescription may be outsourced to another pharmacy; **and**
- Give the name of that pharmacy
    - If the pharmacy is part of a network of pharmacies under common ownership and any of the network pharmacies may dispense the prescription, the patient shall be notified of this

fact. Such notification may be provided through a one-time written notice to the patient or through use of a sign in the pharmacy
- If the prescription is delivered directly to the patient by the dispensing pharmacy and not returned to the requesting pharmacy, place on the prescription container or on a separate sheet delivered with the prescription container, in both English and Spanish, the local, and if applicable, the toll-free telephone number of the pharmacy and the statement: "Written information about this prescription has been provided for you. Please read this information before you take the medication. If you have questions concerning this prescription, a pharmacist is available during normal business hours to answer these questions at [insert the pharmacy's local and toll-free telephone numbers]."

Prescription Labeling

The dispensing pharmacy shall
- Place on the prescription label:
  o Name and address or name and pharmacy license number of the pharmacy dispensing the prescription
  o Name and address of the pharmacy which receives the dispensed prescription
- Indicate in some manner which pharmacy dispensed the prescription (e.g., "Filled by ABC Pharmacy for XYZ Pharmacy")
- Comply with all other labeling requirements

Records

Records may be maintained in an alternative data retention system, such as a data processing system or direct imaging system, provided

- The records contain all of the information required on the manual record; **and**
- The system is capable of producing a hard copy of the record if requested

The requesting pharmacy shall maintain records which indicate the date

- The request for dispensing was transmitted to the dispensing pharmacy; **and**
- The dispensed prescription was received by the requesting pharmacy, including the method of delivery (e.g., private, common, or contract carrier) and the name of the person accepting delivery

The dispensing pharmacy shall maintain records which indicate

- The date the prescription was shipped to the requesting pharmacy
- The name and address where the prescription was shipped
- The method of delivery (e.g., private, common, or contract carrier)

Section Twenty-Eight: Compounding Non-Sterile Preparations

Pharmacies compounding non-sterile preparations, prepackaging pharmaceutical products, and distributing those products shall comply with all requirements for their specific license classification and this section. The purpose of this section is to provide standards for the

- Compounding of non-sterile preparations pursuant to a prescription or medication order for a patient from a practitioner in Class A, Class C, and Class E pharmacies
- Compounding, dispensing, and delivery of a reasonable quantity of a compounded non-sterile preparation in a Class A, Class C, or Class E pharmacy to a practitioner's office for office use by the practitioner
- Compounding and distribution of compounded non-sterile preparations by a Class A pharmacy for a Class C pharmacy
- Compounding of non-sterile preparations by a Class C pharmacy and the distribution of the compounded preparations to other Class C pharmacies under common ownership

Personnel

- All personnel involved in non-sterile compounding must possess the education, training, and proficiency necessary to properly and safely perform compounding duties undertaken or supervised

- A pharmacist shall inspect and approve all components, drug product containers, closures, labeling, and any other materials involved in the compounding process
- A pharmacist shall review all compounding records for accuracy and conduct during and after the compounding process to ensure that errors have not occurred
- All pharmacy technicians and pharmacy technician trainees engaged in non-sterile compounding shall perform compounding duties under the direct supervision of—and responsible to—a pharmacist

Operational Standards

Non-sterile drug preparations may be compounded in licensed pharmacies
- Upon presentation of a practitioner's prescription drug or medication order based on a valid pharmacist/patient/prescriber relationship
- In anticipation of future prescription drug or medication orders based on routine, regularly observed prescribing patterns
- In reasonable quantities for office use by a practitioner and for use by a veterinarian.

Non-sterile compounding in anticipation of future prescription drug or medication orders must be based upon a history of receiving valid prescriptions issued within an established pharmacist/patient/prescriber relationship, provided that in the pharmacist's professional judgment the quantity prepared will be stable for the anticipated shelf time.
- Documentation of the criteria used to determine the stability for the anticipated shelf time must be maintained and be available for inspection

- Any preparation compounded in anticipation of future prescription drug or medication orders shall be labeled
  - Name and strength of the compounded preparation or list of the active ingredients and strengths
  - Facility's lot number
  - Beyond-use date
  - Quantity or amount in the container

Commercially available products may be compounded for dispensing to individual patients, provided the following conditions are met:
- Commercial product is not reasonably available from normal distribution channels in a timely manner to meet patients' needs
- Pharmacy maintains documentation that the product is not reasonably available due to a drug shortage or unavailability from the manufacturer
- Prescribing practitioner has requested that the drug be compounded, as described below
  - Prescribing practitioner shall provide documentation of a patient-specific medical need, and the preparation produces a clinically significant therapeutic response or the drug product is not commercially available
  - Unavailability of such drug product must be documented prior to compounding by a copy of the wholesaler's notification showing back-ordered, discontinued, or out-of-stock items

Other Compounding Rules
- Copies of commercially available products (ex: strength only slightly different) **not** allowed unless practitioner specifically orders the strength or dosage form and

specifies why the patient needs the particular strength or dosage form of the preparation
- A pharmacy may enter into an agreement to compound and dispense prescription/medication orders for another pharmacy, provided the pharmacy complies with the provisions of the title relating to Centralized Prescription Dispensing
- Compounding pharmacies/pharmacists may advertise and promote the fact that they provide non-sterile prescription compounding services, which may include specific drug products and classes of drugs
- A pharmacy may not compound veterinary preparations for use in food-producing animals except in accordance with federal guidelines

Flavoring

- A pharmacist may add flavoring to a prescription at the request of a patient, the patient's agent, or the prescriber
- Pharmacist shall label the flavored prescription with a beyond-use date that shall be no longer than fourteen (14) days if stored in a refrigerator unless otherwise documented
- May **not** add flavoring to an over-the-counter product at the request of a patient or patient's agent unless the pharmacist obtains a prescription for the over-the-counter product from the patient's practitioner

Library

In addition to the library requirements of the pharmacy's specific license classification, a pharmacy shall maintain a current copy, in hard copy or soft copy, of Chapter 795 of the

USP/NF concerning Pharmacy Compounding Non-Sterile Preparations

Environment

- Must have a designated and adequate area for the safe and orderly compounding of non-sterile preparations, including the placement of equipment and materials
- Sink with hot and cold running water, exclusive of rest room facilities, shall be accessible to the compounding areas and be maintained in a sanitary condition

Equipment and Supplies

- Class A prescription balance, or analytical balance and weights, which shall be properly maintained and subject to periodic inspection by the board
- Equipment and utensils necessary for the proper compounding of prescription drug or medication orders

Labeling

In addition to the labeling requirements of the pharmacy's specific license classification, the label dispensed or distributed pursuant to a prescription drug or medication order shall contain the following:

- Generic name(s) or the official name(s) of the principal active ingredient(s) of the compounded preparation
- Statement that the preparation has been compounded by the pharmacy (an auxiliary label may be used on the container to meet this requirement)
- Beyond-use date after which the compounded preparation should not be used

Beyond-Use Date

The beyond-use date shall be determined as outlined in Chapter 795 of the USP/NF concerning Pharmacy Compounding Non-Sterile Preparations including the following

- The pharmacist shall consider
  - Physical and chemical properties of active ingredients
  - Use of preservatives and/or stabilizing agents
  - Dosage form
  - Storage containers and conditions
  - Scientific, laboratory, or reference data from a peer-reviewed source and retained in the pharmacy. The reference data should follow the same preparation instructions for combining raw materials and packaged in a container with similar properties

In the absence of stability information applicable for a specific drug or preparation, the following maximum beyond-use dates are to be used when the compounded preparation is packaged in tight, light-resistant containers and stored at controlled room temperatures

- Nonaqueous liquids and solid formulations (where the manufactured drug product is the source of active ingredient): 25% of the time remaining until the product's expiration date or 6 months, whichever is earlier
- Water-containing formulations (prepared from ingredients in solid form): not later than 14 days when refrigerated between 2–8 degrees Celsius (36–46 degrees Fahrenheit)
- All other formulations: Intended duration of therapy or 30 days, whichever is earlier

Beyond-use date limits may be exceeded when supported by valid scientific stability information for the specific compounded preparation.

Written Drug Information

Written information about the compounded preparation or its major active ingredient(s) shall be given to the patient at the time of dispensing. A statement which indicates that the preparation was compounded by the pharmacy must be included in this written information. If there is no written information available, the patient should be advised that the drug has been compounded and how to contact a pharmacist—and, if appropriate, the prescriber—concerning the drug.

Drugs, Components, and Materials

- Drugs used in non-sterile compounding shall be a USP/NF grade substances manufactured in an FDA-registered facility
- If USP/NF grade substances are not available—or when food, cosmetics, or other substances are, or must be used—the substance shall be of a chemical grade in one of the following categories
  - Chemically Pure (CP)
  - Analytical Reagent (AR)
  - American Chemical Society (ACS)
  - Food Chemical Codex
- A manufactured drug product may be a source of active ingredient. Only manufactured drugs from containers labeled with a batch control number and a future expiration date are acceptable as a potential source of active ingredients
- All components shall be stored in properly labeled containers in a clean, dry area, under proper temperatures

- Drug product containers and closures shall not be reactive, additive, or absorptive so as to alter the safety, identity, strength, quality, or purity of the compounded drug product beyond the desired result
- A pharmacy may not compound a preparation that contains ingredients appearing on a federal Food and Drug Administration list of drug products withdrawn or removed from the market for safety reasons

Compounding Process

- Standard operating procedures must be in place
- Any compounded preparation with an official monograph in the USP/NF shall be compounded, labeled, and packaged in conformity with the USP/NF monograph for the drug
- Any person with an apparent illness or open lesion that may adversely affect the safety or quality of a drug product being compounded shall be excluded from direct contact with components, drug product containers, closures, any materials involved in the compounding process, and drug products until the condition is corrected
- Personnel engaged in the compounding of drug preparations shall wear clean clothing appropriate to the operation being performed. Protective apparel—such as coats/jackets, aprons, hair nets, gowns, hand or arm coverings, or masks—shall be worn as necessary to protect personnel from chemical exposure and drug preparations from contamination
- At each step of the compounding process, the pharmacist shall ensure that components used in compounding are accurately weighed, measured, or subdivided as appropriate to conform to the formula being prepared

Quality Assurance

Initial formula validation

- Prior to routine compounding of a non-sterile preparation, a pharmacy shall conduct an evaluation that shows that the pharmacy is capable of compounding a product that contains the stated amount of active ingredient(s)

Finished preparation checks

- The prescription drug and medication orders, written compounding procedure, preparation records, and expended materials used to make compounded non-sterile preparations shall be inspected for accuracy of correct identities and amounts of ingredients, packaging, labeling, and expected physical appearance before the non-sterile preparations are dispensed

Quality Control

- The pharmacy shall follow established quality control procedures to monitor the quality of compounded drug preparations for uniformity and consistency such as capsule weight variations, adequacy of mixing, clarity, or pH of solutions
- Compounding procedures that are routinely performed, including batch compounding, shall be completed and verified according to written procedures. The act of verification of a compounding procedure involves checking to ensure that calculations, weighing and measuring, order of mixing, and compounding techniques were appropriate and accurately performed
- Unless otherwise indicated or appropriate, compounded preparations are to be prepared to ensure that each preparation shall contain not less than 90.0% and not more than 110.0% of the theoretically

calculated and labeled quantity of active ingredient per unit weight or volume and not less than 90.0% and not more than 110.0% of the theoretically calculated weight or volume per unit of the preparation

Office Use Compounding and Distribution of Compounded Preparations to Class C Pharmacies or Veterinarians

- A pharmacy may dispense and deliver a reasonable quantity of a compounded preparation to a practitioner for office use by the practitioner
- A Class A pharmacy is not required to register or be licensed under Chapter 431, Health and Safety Code, to distribute non-sterile compounded preparations to a Class C pharmacy
- A Class C pharmacy is not required to register or be licensed under Chapter 431, Health and Safety Code, to distribute non-sterile compounded preparations that the Class C pharmacy has compounded for other Class C pharmacies under common ownership
- To dispense and deliver a compounded preparation under this subsection, a pharmacy must
    - o Verify the source of the raw materials to be used in a compounded drug
    - o Comply with applicable USP guidelines, including the testing requirements
    - o Enter into a written agreement with a practitioner for the practitioner's office use of a compounded preparation
    - o Comply with all applicable competency and accrediting standards as determined by the board

Recall Procedures

- The pharmacy shall have written procedures for the recall of any compounded non-sterile preparations provided to a patient, to a practitioner for office use, or a pharmacy for administration. Written procedures shall include, but not be limited to the requirements as specified in this section
- The pharmacy shall immediately initiate a recall of any non-sterile preparation compounded by the pharmacy upon identification of a potential or confirmed harm to a patient
- In the event of a recall, the pharmacist-in-charge shall ensure that:
    - Each practitioner, facility, and/or pharmacy to which the preparation was distributed is notified, in writing, of the recall
    - Each patient to whom the preparation was dispensed is notified, in writing, of the recall
    - If the preparation is prepared as a batch, the board is notified of the recall, in writing
    - If the preparation is distributed for office use, the Texas Department of State Health Services, Drugs and Medical Devices Group, is notified of the recall, in writing
    - The preparation is quarantined
    - The pharmacy keeps a written record of the recall including all actions taken to notify all parties and steps taken to ensure corrective measures
- If a pharmacy fails to initiate a recall, the board may require a pharmacy to initiate a recall if there is potential for or confirmed harm to a patient

Section Twenty-Nine: Compounding Sterile Preparations

Pharmacies compounding sterile preparations, prepackaging pharmaceutical products, and distributing those products shall comply with all requirements for their specific license classification and this section. The purpose of this section is to provide standards for the

- Compounding of sterile preparations pursuant to a prescription or medication order for a patient from a practitioner in Class A-S, Class B, Class C-S, and Class E-S pharmacies
- Compounding, dispensing, and delivery of a reasonable quantity of a compounded sterile preparation in a Class A-S, Class B, Class C-S, and Class E-S pharmacies to a practitioner's office for office use by the practitioner
- Compounding and distribution of compounded sterile preparations by a Class A-S pharmacy for a Class C-S pharmacy
- Compounding of sterile preparations by a Class C-S pharmacy and the distribution of the compounded preparations to other Class C or Class C-S pharmacies under common ownership

Pharmacist-In-Charge
- Pharmacy shall have a PIC in compliance with the specific license classification of the pharmacy
- In addition to the responsibilities for the specific class of pharmacy, the PIC shall have the responsibility for, at a minimum, the following concerning the compounding of sterile preparations:

285

- Developing a system to ensure that all pharmacy personnel responsible for compounding and/or supervising the compounding of sterile preparations within the pharmacy receive appropriate education and training and competency evaluation
- Determining that all personnel involved in compounding sterile preparations obtain continuing education appropriate for the type of compounding done by the personnel
- Supervising a system to ensure appropriate procurement of drugs and devices and storage of all pharmaceutical materials including pharmaceuticals, components used in the compounding of sterile preparations, and drug delivery devices
- Ensuring that the equipment used in compounding is properly maintained
- Developing a system for the disposal and distribution of drugs from the pharmacy
- Developing a system for bulk compounding or batch preparation of drugs
- Developing a system for the compounding, sterility assurance, quality assurance, and quality control of sterile preparations
- If applicable, ensuring that the pharmacy has a system to dispose of hazardous waste in a manner so as not to endanger the public health

Pharmacists

- Responsible for ensuring that compounded sterile preparations are accurately identified, measured, diluted, and mixed and are correctly purified, sterilized, packaged, sealed, labeled, stored, dispensed, and distributed

- Inspect and approve all components, drug preparation containers, closures, labeling, and any other materials involved in the compounding process
- Review all compounding records for accuracy and conduct in-process and final checks and verification of calculations to ensure that errors have not occurred in the compounding process
- Responsible for ensuring the proper maintenance, cleanliness, and use of all equipment used in the compounding process
- Accessible at all times, 24 hours a day, to respond to patients' and other health professionals' questions and needs

Pharmacist Training Prior to September 1, 2015

Prior to September 1, 2015 - initial training and continuing education

- All pharmacists who compound sterile preparations for administration to patients or supervise pharmacy technicians and pharmacy technician trainees compounding sterile preparations shall:
  - Complete through a single course, a minimum of 20 hours of instruction and experience in the areas listed in "Evaluation and Testing Requirements" section. Such training may be obtained through either:
    - Completion of a structured on-the-job didactic and experiential training program at this pharmacy which provides 20 hours of instruction and experience. Such training may not be transferred to another pharmacy unless the pharmacies are under common ownership and control and use a common training program; OR

- Completion of a recognized course in an accredited college of pharmacy or a course sponsored by an ACPE accredited provider which provides 20 hours of instruction and experience
  - o Possess knowledge about:
    - Aseptic processing
    - Quality control and quality assurance as related to environmental, component, and finished preparation release checks and tests
    - Chemical, pharmaceutical, and clinical properties of drugs
    - Container, equipment, and closure system selection
    - Sterilization techniques
- The required experiential portion of the training programs specified in this subparagraph must be supervised by an individual who has already completed training
- Complete continuing education related to the type of compounding done

Pharmacist Training Effective September 1, 2015

Effective September 1, 2015 - initial training and continuing education

- All pharmacists who compound sterile preparations or supervise pharmacy technicians and pharmacy technician trainees compounding sterile preparations shall comply with the following:
  - o Complete through a single course, a minimum of 20 hours of instruction and experience in the areas listed in "Evaluation and Testing Requirements" section. Such training shall be obtained through completion of a recognized

course in an accredited college of pharmacy or a course sponsored by an ACPE accredited provider
- o Complete a structured on-the-job didactic and experiential training program at this pharmacy which provides sufficient hours of instruction and experience in the facility's sterile compounding processes and procedures. Such training may not be transferred to another pharmacy unless the pharmacies are under common ownership and control and use a common training program; and
- o Possess knowledge about:
  - aseptic processing
  - Quality control and quality assurance as related to environmental, component, and finished preparation release checks and tests
  - Chemical, pharmaceutical, and clinical properties of drugs
  - Container, equipment, and closure system selection
  - Sterilization techniques
- The required experiential portion of the training programs specified in this subparagraph must be supervised by an individual who is actively engaged in performing sterile compounding and is qualified and has completed training as specified in this section
- In order to renew a license to practice pharmacy, during the previous licensure period, a pharmacist engaged in sterile compounding shall complete a minimum of:
  - o Two hours of ACPE-accredited continuing education relating to one or more of the areas listed in "Evaluation and Testing Requirements" section if the pharmacist is engaged in

compounding low and medium risk sterile preparations; OR

- o Four hours of ACPE-accredited continuing education relating to one or more of the areas listed in "Evaluation and Testing Requirements" section if the pharmacist is engaged in compounding high risk sterile preparations

Pharmacy Technicians and Pharmacy Technician Trainees Training Prior to September 1, 2015

Prior to September 1, 2015 - initial training and continuing education. In addition to specific qualifications for registration, all pharmacy technicians and pharmacy technician trainees who compound sterile preparations for administration to patients shall:

- Have initial training obtained either through completion of:
  - o A single course, a minimum of 40 hours of instruction and experience in the areas listed in "Evaluation and Testing Requirements" section. Such training may be obtained through:
    - Completion of a structured on-the-job didactic and experiential training program at this pharmacy which provides 40 hours of instruction and experience. Such training may not be transferred to another pharmacy unless the pharmacies are under common ownership and control and use a common training program; OR
    - Completion of a course sponsored by an ACPE accredited provider which provides 40 hours of instruction and experience; OR

- A training program which is accredited by the American Society of Health-System Pharmacists. Individuals enrolled in training programs accredited by the American Society of Health-System Pharmacists may compound sterile preparations in a licensed pharmacy provided:
    - The compounding occurs only during times the individual is assigned to a pharmacy as a part of the experiential component of the American Society of Health-System Pharmacists training program
    - The individual is under the direct supervision of and responsible to a pharmacist who has completed training
    - The supervising pharmacist conducts in-process and final checks
- Acquire the required experiential portion of the training programs specified in this subparagraph under the supervision of an individual who has already completed training as specified

Pharmacy Technicians and Pharmacy Technician Trainees Training Effective September 1, 2015

Effective September 1, 2015 - initial training and continuing education

- Pharmacy technicians and pharmacy technician trainees may compound sterile preparations provided the pharmacy technicians and/or pharmacy technician trainees are supervised by a pharmacist who has completed the training, conducts in-process and final checks, and affixes his or her initials to the appropriate quality control records

- All pharmacy technicians and pharmacy technician trainees who compound sterile preparations for administration to patients shall comply with the following:
    - Complete through completion of a single course, a minimum of 40 hours of instruction and experience in the areas listed in "Evaluation and Testing Requirements" section. Such training shall be obtained through completion of a course sponsored by an ACPE accredited provider which provides 40 hours of instruction and experience
    - Complete a structured on-the-job didactic and experiential training program at this pharmacy which provides sufficient hours of instruction and experience in the facility's sterile compounding processes and procedures the areas. Such training may not be transferred to another pharmacy unless the pharmacies are under common ownership and control and use a common training program; and
    - Possess knowledge about:
        - Aseptic processing
        - Quality control and quality assurance as related to environmental, component, and finished preparation release checks and tests
        - Chemical, pharmaceutical, and clinical properties of drugs
        - Container, equipment, and closure system selection
        - Sterilization techniques
- Individuals enrolled in training programs accredited by the American Society of Health-System Pharmacists

may compound sterile preparations in a licensed
pharmacy provided:
- o Compounding occurs only during times the
  individual is assigned to a pharmacy as a part of
  the experiential component of the American
  Society of Health-System Pharmacists training
  program
- o Individual is under the direct supervision of and
  responsible to a pharmacist who has the
  completed training
- o Supervising pharmacist conducts in-process and
  final checks
- The required experiential portion of the training
  programs must be supervised by an individual who is
  actively engaged in performing sterile compounding, is
  qualified and has completed the training
- In order to renew a registration as a pharmacy
  technician, during the previous registration period, a
  pharmacy technician engaged in sterile compounding
  shall complete a minimum of:
  - o Two hours of ACPE accredited continuing
    education relating to one or more of the areas
    listed in "Evaluation and Testing Requirements"
    section if the pharmacy technician is engaged in
    compounding low and medium risk sterile
    preparations; OR
  - o Four hours of ACPE accredited continuing
    education relating to one or more of the areas
    listed in "Evaluation and Testing Requirements"
    section if pharmacy technician is engaged in
    compounding high risk sterile preparations

Evaluation and Testing Requirements

- All pharmacy personnel preparing sterile preparations shall be trained conscientiously and skillfully by expert personnel through multimedia instructional sources and professional publications in the theoretical principles and practical skills of aseptic manipulations, garbing procedures, aseptic work practices, achieving and maintaining ISO Class 5 environmental conditions, and cleaning and disinfection procedures before beginning to prepare compounded sterile preparations
- All pharmacy personnel preparing sterile preparations shall perform didactic review and pass written and media-fill testing of aseptic manipulative skills initially followed by:
  - Every 12 months for low- and medium-risk level compounding
  - Every six months for high-risk level compounding
- Pharmacy personnel who fail written tests or whose media-fill test vials result in gross microbial colonization shall:
  - Be immediately re-instructed and re-evaluated by expert compounding personnel to ensure correction of all aseptic practice deficiencies; and
  - Not be allowed to compound sterile preparations for patient use until passing results are achieved
- The didactic and experiential training shall include instruction, experience, and demonstrated proficiency in the following areas:
  - Aseptic technique
  - Critical area contamination factors
  - Environmental monitoring
  - Structure and engineering controls related to facilities
  - Equipment and supplies

- o Sterile preparation calculations and terminology
  - o Sterile preparation compounding documentation
  - o Quality assurance procedures
  - o Aseptic preparation procedures including proper gowning and gloving technique
  - o Handling of hazardous drugs, if applicable
  - o Cleaning procedures
  - o General conduct in the clean room
- The aseptic technique of each person compounding or responsible for the direct supervision of personnel compounding sterile preparations shall be observed and evaluated by expert personnel as satisfactory through written and practical tests, and media-fill challenge testing, and such evaluation documented
- Media-fill tests must be conducted at each pharmacy where an individual compounds sterile preparations. No preparation intended for patient use shall be compounded by an individual until the on-site media-fill tests indicate that the individual can competently perform aseptic procedures, except that a pharmacist may temporarily compound sterile preparations and supervise pharmacy technicians compounding sterile preparations without media-fill tests provided the pharmacist completes the on-site media-fill tests within seven days of commencing work at the pharmacy
- Media-fill tests procedures for assessing the preparation of specific types of sterile preparations shall be representative of the most challenging or stressful conditions encountered by the pharmacy personnel being evaluated for each risk level and for sterilizing high-risk level compounded sterile preparations
- Media-fill challenge tests simulating high-risk level compounding shall be used to verify the capability of

the compounding environment and process to produce a sterile preparation
- Commercially available sterile fluid culture media, such as Soybean-Casein Digest Medium shall be able to promote exponential colonization of bacteria that are most likely to be transmitted to compounding sterile preparations from the compounding personnel and environment. Media-filled vials are generally incubated at 20 to 25 or at 30 to 35 for a minimum of 14 days. If two temperatures are used for incubation of media-filled samples, then these filled containers should be incubated for at least 7 days at each temperature. Failure is indicated by visible turbidity in the medium on or before 14 days
- PIC shall ensure continuing competency of pharmacy personnel through in-service education, training, and media-fill tests to supplement initial training. Personnel competency shall be evaluated:
  - During orientation and training prior to the regular performance of those tasks
  - Whenever the quality assurance program yields an unacceptable result
  - Whenever unacceptable techniques are observed
  - At least on an annual basis for low- and medium-risk level compounding, and every six months for high-risk level compounding
- The pharmacist-in-charge shall ensure that proper hand hygiene and garbing practices of compounding personnel are evaluated prior to compounding sterile preparations intended for patient use and whenever an aseptic media fill is performed
  - Sampling of compounding personnel glove fingertips shall be performed for all risk level compounding

- All compounding personnel shall demonstrate competency in proper hand hygiene and garbing procedures and in aseptic work practices (e.g., disinfection of component surfaces, routine disinfection of gloved hands)
- Sterile contact agar plates shall be used to sample the gloved fingertips of compounding personnel after garbing in order to assess garbing competency and after completing the media-fill preparation (without applying sterile 70% IPA)
- The visual observation shall be documented and maintained to provide a permanent record and long-term assessment of personnel competency
- All compounding personnel shall successfully complete an initial competency evaluation and gloved fingertip/thumb sampling procedure no less than three times before initially being allowed to compound sterile preparations for patient use. Immediately after the compounding personnel completes the hand hygiene and garbing procedure (e.g., donning of sterile gloves prior to any disinfection with sterile 70% IPA), the evaluator will collect a gloved fingertip and thumb sample from both hands from the compounding personnel onto agar plates by lightly pressing each fingertip into the agar. The plates will be incubated for the appropriate incubation period and at the appropriate temperature. Re-evaluation of all compounding personnel shall occur at least annually for compounding personnel who compound low and medium risk level preparations and every six months for compounding personnel who compound high risk level preparations.

- The pharmacist-in-charge shall ensure surface sampling shall be conducted in all ISO classified areas on a periodic basis. Sampling shall be accomplished using contact plates at the conclusion of compounding. The sample area shall be gently touched with the agar surface by rolling the plate across the surface to be sampled

Documentation of Training

The pharmacy shall maintain a record of the training and continuing education on each person who compounds sterile preparations. The record shall contain, at a minimum, a written record of initial and in-service training, education, and the results of written and practical testing and media-fill testing of pharmacy personnel. The record shall be maintained and available for inspection by the board and contain the following information:

- Name of the person receiving the training or completing the testing or media-fill tests
- Date(s) of the training, testing, or media-fill challenge testing
- General description of the topics covered in the training or testing or of the process validated
- Name of the person supervising the training, testing, or media-fill challenge testing
- Signature or initials of the person receiving the training or completing the testing or media-fill challenge testing and the pharmacist-in-charge or other pharmacist employed by the pharmacy and designated by the pharmacist-in-charge as responsible for training, testing, or media-fill challenge testing of personnel

Operational Standards

Sterile preparations may be compounded in licensed pharmacies

- Upon presentation of a practitioner's prescription drug or medication order based on a valid pharmacist/patient/prescriber relationship
- In anticipation of future prescription drug or medication orders based on routine, regularly observed prescribing patterns (see more on this under non-sterile compounding)
- In reasonable quantities for office use by a practitioner and for use by a veterinarian

Any preparation compounded in anticipation of future prescription drug or medication orders shall be labeled

- Name and strength of the compounded preparation **or** list of the active ingredients and strengths
- Facility's lot number
- Beyond-use date
- Quantity or amount in the container
- Appropriate ancillary instructions, such as storage instructions or cautionary statements, including hazardous drug warning labels where appropriate

Other Rules

- Commercially available products – same conditions as non-sterile compounding
- A pharmacy may enter into an agreement to compound and dispense prescription/medication orders for another pharmacy, provided the pharmacy complies with the title relating to Centralized Prescription Dispensing

- Compounding pharmacies/pharmacists may advertise and promote the fact that they provide sterile prescription compounding services, which may include specific drug preparations and classes of drugs
- A pharmacy may not compound veterinary preparations for use in food-producing animals except in accordance with federal guidelines

Microbial Contamination Risk Levels

Risk Levels for sterile compounded preparations shall be as outlined in Chapter 797, Pharmacy Compounding—Sterile Preparations of the USP/NF and as listed below

Low-risk level compounded sterile preparations

- The compounded sterile preparations are compounded with aseptic manipulations entirely within ISO Class 5 or better air quality using only sterile ingredients, products, components, and devices
- The compounding involves only transfer, measuring, and mixing manipulations with closed or sealed packaging systems that are preformed promptly and attentively
- Manipulations are limited to aseptically opening ampules, penetrating sterile stoppers on vials with sterile needles and syringes, and transferring sterile liquids in sterile syringes to sterile administration devices and packages of other sterile products
- For a low-risk preparation, the storage periods may not exceed the following periods before administration:
  - 48 hours at controlled room temperature
  - 14 days if stored at a cold temperature
  - 45 days if stored in a frozen state, at minus 20 degrees Celsius or colder

300

- For delayed activation device systems, the storage period begins when the device is activated

Examples of Low-Risk Compounding

- Single volume transfers of sterile dosage forms from ampules, bottles, bags, and vials; using sterile syringes with sterile needles, other administration devices, and other sterile containers
- Manually measuring and mixing no more than *three (3)* manufactured products to compound drug admixtures

Low-Risk Level compounded sterile preparations with 12-hour or fewer beyond-use date

- The compounded sterile preparations are compounded in compounding aseptic isolator or compounding aseptic containment isolator that is not ISO Class 5 or better or the compounded sterile preparations are compounded in laminar airflow workbench or a biological safety cabinet that cannot be located within an ISO Class 7 buffer area
- Administration of such compounded sterile preparations must commence within 12 hours of preparation or as recommended in the manufacturers' package insert, whichever is less

Medium-risk level compounded sterile preparations

Medium-risk level compounded sterile preparations are those compounded aseptically under low-risk conditions, and one or more of the following conditions exist

- Multiple individual or small doses of sterile products are combined or pooled to prepare a compounded sterile preparation that will be administered either to multiple patients or to one patient on multiple occasions

- The compounding process includes complex aseptic manipulations other than the single-volume transfer
- The compounding process requires unusually long duration, such as that required to complete the dissolution or homogenous mixing (e.g., reconstitution of intravenous immunoglobulin or other intravenous protein products)
- The compounded sterile preparations do not contain broad-spectrum bacteriostatic substances and they are administered over several days (e.g., an externally worn infusion device)
- For a medium-risk preparation, the beyond-use dates may not exceed the following time periods before administration:
  - 30 hours at controlled room temperature
  - 9 days at a cold temperature
  - 45 days in solid frozen state, at minus 20 degrees Celsius or colder

Examples of medium-risk compounding

- Compounding of total parenteral nutrition fluids using a manual or automated device, during which there are multiple injections, detachments, and attachments of nutrient-source products to the device or machine to deliver all nutritional components to a final sterile container
- Filling of reservoirs of injection and infusion devices with multiple sterile drug products, and evacuating air from those reservoirs before the filled device is dispensed
- Filling of reservoirs of injection and infusion devices with volumes of sterile drug solutions that will be administered over several days at ambient

temperatures between 25 and 40 degrees Celsius (77 and 104 degrees Fahrenheit)
- Transferring volumes from multiple ampules or vials into a single, final sterile container or product

High-risk level compounded sterile preparations

High-risk level compounded sterile preparations are those compounded under any of the following conditions
- Non-sterile ingredients, including manufactured products, are incorporated; or a non-sterile device is employed before terminal sterilization
- Sterile ingredients, components, devices, and mixtures are exposed to air quality inferior to ISO Class 5.
  - This includes storage in environments inferior to ISO Class 5 of opened or partially used packages of manufactured sterile products that lack antimicrobial preservatives
- Non-sterile preparations are exposed no more than 6 hours before being sterilized
- For a high-risk preparation, the beyond-use dates may not exceed the following time periods before administration:
  - 24 hours at controlled room temperature
  - 3 days at a cold temperature
  - 45 days in solid frozen state, at minus 20 degrees or colder
- All high-risk compounded sterile aqueous solutions subjected to terminal sterilization are passed through a filter with a nominal porosity not larger than 1.2 micron preceding or during filling into their final containers to remove particulate matter. Sterilization of high-risk level compounded sterile preparations by filtration shall be performed entirely within an ISO Class 5 or superior air quality environment

Examples of high-risk compounding
- Dissolving non-sterile bulk drug powders to make solutions, which will be terminally sterilized
- Exposing the sterile ingredients and components used to prepare and package compounded sterile preparations to room air quality worse than ISO Class 5
- Measuring and mixing sterile ingredients in non-sterile devices before sterilization is performed
- Assuming, without appropriate evidence or direct determination, that packages of bulk ingredients contain at least 95% by weight of their active chemical moiety and have not been contaminated or adulterated between uses

Immediate Use Compounded Sterile Preparations

For the purpose of emergency or immediate patient care, such situations may include cardiopulmonary resuscitation, emergency room treatment, preparation of diagnostic agents, or critical therapy where the preparation of the compounded sterile preparation under low-risk level conditions would subject the patient to additional risk due to delays in therapy. Compounded sterile preparations are exempted from the requirements described in this paragraph for low-risk, medium-risk, and high-risk level compounded sterile preparations when all of the following criteria are met.
- Only simple aseptic measuring and transfer manipulations are performed with not more than three (3) sterile non-hazardous commercial drug and diagnostic radiopharmaceutical drug products, including an infusion or diluent solution
- Unless required for the preparation, the preparation procedure occurs continuously without delays or interruptions and does not exceed 1 hour

- Administration begins not later than one (1) hour following the completion of preparing the compounded sterile preparation
- When the compounded sterile preparations is not administered by the person who prepared it or its administration is not witnessed by the person who prepared it, the compounded sterile preparation shall bear a label listing patient identification information such as name and identification number(s), the names and amounts of all ingredients, the name or initials of the person who prepared the compounded sterile preparation, and the exact 1-hour beyond-use time and date
- If administration has not begun within one (1) hour following the completion of preparing the compounded sterile preparation, the compounded sterile preparation is promptly and safely discarded. Immediate-use compounded sterile preparations shall not be stored for later use
- Cytotoxic drugs shall not be prepared as immediate-use compounded sterile preparations

Single-Dose and Multiple Dose Containers

- Opened or needle punctured single-dose containers, such as bags bottles, syringes, and vials of sterile products shall be used within one hour if opened in worse than ISO Class 5 air quality. Any remaining contents must be discarded
- Single-dose containers, including single-dose large volume parenteral solutions and single-dose vials, exposed to ISO Class 5 or cleaner air may be used up to six hours after initial needle puncture
- Opened single-dose fusion sealed containers shall not be stored for any time period

- Multiple-dose containers may be used up to 28 days after initial needle puncture unless otherwise specified by the manufacturer

Library

In addition to the library requirements of the pharmacy's specific license classification, a pharmacy shall maintain current or updated copies in physical or electronic format of each of the following
- Reference text on injectable drug preparations, such as Handbook on Injectable Drug Products
- Specialty reference text appropriate for the scope of pharmacy services provided by the pharmacy, e.g., if the pharmacy prepares hazardous drugs, a reference text on the preparation of hazardous drugs
- United States Pharmacopeia/National Formulary or the USP Pharmacist's Pharmacopeia containing USP Chapter 797, Pharmaceutical Compounding—Sterile Preparations

Environment

A pharmacy that prepares low- and medium-risk preparations shall have a clean room/controlled area for the compounding of sterile preparations that is constructed to minimize the opportunities for particulate and microbial contamination. The clean room/controlled area shall
- Contain an anteroom/ante-zone that provides at least an ISO Class 8 air quality
- Contain a buffer zone or buffer room designed to maintain at least ISO Class 7 conditions

The pharmacy shall prepare sterile pharmaceuticals in a primary engineering control device, such as a laminar air flow hood, biological safety cabinet, compounding aseptic isolator,

306

compounding aseptic containment isolator which is capable of maintaining at least ISO Class 5 conditions during normal activity. The isolator must provide isolation from the room and maintain ISO Class 5 during dynamic operating conditions, including transferring ingredients, components, and devices into and out of the isolator and during preparation of compounded sterile preparations

Cytotoxic Drugs

- All personnel involved in the compounding of cytotoxic products shall wear appropriate protective apparel, such as gowns, face masks, eye protection, hair covers, shoe covers or dedicated shoes, and appropriate gloving
- Cytotoxic drugs shall be prepared in a Class II or III vertical flow biological safety cabinet or compounding aseptic containment isolator located in an ISO Class 7 area that is physically separated from other preparation areas
- Compounding area must have negative air pressure compared to the anteroom, which must have positive air pressure
- Hazardous drugs shall be stored separately from other inventory in a manner to prevent contamination and personnel exposure

Cleaning and Disinfecting the Sterile Compounding Areas

- Shall be conducted at the beginning of each work shift, before each batch preparation is started, every 30 minutes during continuous compounding of individual compounded sterile preparations, when there are spills,

and when surface contamination is known or suspected from procedural breaches
- Before compounding is performed, all items are removed from the direct and contiguous compounding areas and all surfaces are cleaned of loose material and residue from spills, followed by an application of a residue-free disinfecting agent (e.g., IPA), that is left on for a time sufficient to exert its antimicrobial effect
- Work surfaces near the direct and contiguous compounding areas in the buffer or clean area are cleaned of loose material and residue from spills, followed by an application of a residue-free disinfecting agent that is left on for a time sufficient to exert its antimicrobial effect
- Floors in the buffer or clean area are cleaned by mopping at least once daily when no aseptic operations are in progress
- In the buffer area, ante-area, and segregated compounding area, walls, ceilings, and shelving shall be cleaned and disinfected monthly
- Supplies and equipment removed from shipping cartons must be wiped with a disinfecting agent, such as IPA. No shipping or other external cartons may be taken into the buffer or clean area
- Storage shelving, emptied of all supplies, walls, and ceilings are cleaned and disinfected at least monthly

Equipment and Supplies

Pharmacies compounding sterile preparations shall have the following equipment and supplies:
- A calibrated system or device (i.e., thermometer) to monitor the temperature to ensure that proper storage requirements are met, if sterile preparations are stored in the refrigerator

- A calibrated system or device to monitor the temperature where bulk chemicals are stored
- A temperature-sensing mechanism suitably placed in the controlled temperature storage space to reflect accurately the true temperature
- If applicable, a Class A prescription balance, or analytical balance and weights. Such balance shall be properly maintained and subject to periodic inspection by the Texas State Board of Pharmacy
- Equipment and utensils necessary for the proper compounding of sterile preparations. Such equipment and utensils used in the compounding process shall be:
    - Of appropriate design, appropriate capacity, and be operated within designed operational limits
    - Of suitable composition so that surfaces that contact components, in-process material, or drug products shall not be reactive, additive, or absorptive so as to alter the safety, identity, strength, quality, or purity of the drug preparation beyond the desired result
    - Cleaned and sanitized immediately prior to and after each use
    - Routinely inspected, calibrated(if necessary), or checked to ensure proper performance
- Appropriate disposal containers for used needles, syringes, etc., and if applicable, hazardous waste from the preparation of hazardous drugs and/or biohazardous waste
- Appropriate packaging or delivery containers to maintain proper storage conditions for sterile preparations
- Infusion devices, if applicable
- All necessary supplies, including:
    - Disposable needles, syringes, and other supplies for aseptic mixing

- o   Disinfectant cleaning solutions
- o   Hand washing agents with bactericidal action
- o   Disposable, lint free towels or wipes
- o   Appropriate filters and filtration equipment
- o   Hazardous spill kits, if applicable
- o   Masks, caps, coveralls or gowns with tight cuffs, shoe covers, and gloves, as applicable

Labeling

In addition to the labeling requirements for the pharmacy's specific license classification, the label dispensed or distributed pursuant to a prescription drug or medication order shall contain the following:

- Generic name(s) or the official name(s) of the principal active ingredient(s) of the compounded sterile preparation
- For outpatient prescription orders only, a statement that the compounded sterile preparation has been compounded by the pharmacy
- Beyond-use date

If the sterile pharmaceutical is compounded in a batch, the following shall also be included on the batch label:

- Unique lot number assigned to the batch
- Quantity
- Appropriate ancillary instructions, such as storage instructions or cautionary statements, including hazardous drug warning labels where appropriate

Personnel Cleansing and Garbing

- Any person with an apparent illness or open lesion that may adversely affect the safety or quality of a drug preparation being compounded shall be excluded from direct contact with components, drug preparation containers, closures, any materials involved in the

compounding process, and drug products until the condition is corrected
- Before entering the clean area, compounding personnel must remove the following:
    o Personal outer garments (e.g., bandanas, coats, hats, jackets, scarves, sweaters, vests)
    o all cosmetics, because they shed flakes and particles; **and**
    o all hand, wrist, and other body jewelry
- Artificial nails or extenders are prohibited while working in the sterile compounding environment
- Personnel must don personal protective equipment and perform hand hygiene in an order that proceeds from the dirtiest to the cleanest activities as follows:
    o Shoe covers
    o Head and facial hair covers
    o Face mask
    o Wash hands and arms up to elbows – minimum 30 seconds
    o Gown
    o Gloves
    o 70% IPA to gloves (and routinely during compounding)
- When taking a break – the gown may be stored in the anteroom and reused, but shoe covers, hair and facial hair covers, face mask, and gloves must be replaced, and hand hygiene must be performed

Finished Preparation Release Checks and Tests
- All high-risk level compounded sterile preparations that are prepared in groups of more than 25 identical individual single-dose packages (such as ampuls, bags, syringes, and vials), or in multiple dose vials for administration to multiple patients, or are exposed longer than 12 hours at 2 - 8 degrees Celsius and longer

311

than six hours at warmer than 8 degrees Celsius before they are sterilized shall be tested to ensure they are sterile and do not contain excessive bacterial endotoxins as specified in Chapter 71, Sterility Tests of the USP/NF before being dispensed or administered
- Visually examine all compounded sterile preparations for particulate matter prior to dispensing and administration
- The prescription drug and medication orders, written compounding procedure, preparation records, and expended materials used to make compounded sterile preparations at all contamination risk levels shall be inspected for accuracy of correct identities and amounts of ingredients, aseptic mixing and sterilization, packaging, labeling, and expected physical appearance before they are dispensed or administered

Viable and Nonviable Environmental Sampling Testing

Environmental sampling shall occur, at a minimum, every six months as part of a comprehensive quality management program and under any of the following conditions:
- As part of the commissioning and certification of new facilities and equipment
- Following any servicing of facilities and equipment
- As part of the re-certification of facilities and equipment
- In response to identified problems with end products or staff technique
- In response to issues with compounded sterile preparations, observed compounding personnel work practices, or patient-related infections (where the compounded sterile preparation is being considered as a potential source of the infection)

Total Particle Counts

Certification that each ISO classified area (e.g., ISO Class 5, 7, and 8), is within established guidelines shall be performed no less than every six months and whenever the equipment is relocated or the physical structure of the buffer area or ante-area has been altered. All certification records shall be maintained and reviewed to ensure that the controlled environments comply with the proper air cleanliness, room pressures, and air changes per hour. Testing shall be performed by qualified operators using current, state-of-the-art equipment, with results of the following:

- ISO Class 5 - not more than 3520 particles 0.5 μm and larger size per cubic meter of air
- ISO Class 7 - not more than 352,000 particles of 0.5 μm and larger size per cubic meter of air for any buffer area
- ISO Class 8 - not more than 3,520,000 particles of 0.5 μm and larger size per cubic meter of air for any ante-area

Pressure Differential Monitoring

A pressure gauge or velocity meter shall be installed to monitor the pressure differential or airflow between the buffer area and the ante-area and between the ante-area and the general environment outside the compounding area. The results shall be reviewed and documented on a log at least every work shift (minimum frequency shall be at least daily) or by a continuous recording device. The pressure between the ISO Class 7 and the general pharmacy area shall not be less than 0.02 inch water column.

Viable Air Sampling

Evaluation of airborne microorganisms using volumetric collection methods in the controlled air environments shall be performed by properly trained individuals for all compounding risk levels. For low-, medium-, and high-risk level compounding, air sampling shall be performed at locations that are prone to contamination during compounding activities and during other activities such as staging, labeling, gowning, and cleaning. Locations shall include zones of air backwash turbulence within the laminar airflow workbench and other areas where air backwash turbulence may enter the compounding area. For low-risk level compounded sterile preparations within 12-hour or less beyond-use-date prepared in a primary engineering control that maintains an ISO Class 5, air sampling shall be performed at locations inside the ISO Class 5 environment and other areas that are in close proximity to the ISO Class 5 environment during the certification of the primary engineering control

Air Sampling Frequency and Process

Air sampling shall be performed at least every 6 months as a part of the re-certification of facilities and equipment. A sufficient volume of air shall be sampled and the manufacturer's guidelines for use of the electronic air sampling equipment followed. At the end of the designated sampling or exposure period for air sampling activities, the microbial growth media plates are recovered and their covers secured and they are inverted and incubated at a temperature and for a time period conducive to multiplication of microorganisms. Sampling data shall be collected and reviewed on a periodic basis as a means of evaluating the overall control of the compounding environment. If an activity consistently shows elevated levels of microbial growth, competent microbiology personnel shall be consulted

Compounding Accuracy Checks

Written procedures for double-checking compounding accuracy shall be followed for every compounded sterile preparation during preparation and immediately prior to release, including label accuracy and the accuracy of the addition of all drug products or ingredients used to prepare the finished preparation and their volumes or quantities. At each step of the compounding process, the pharmacist shall ensure that components used in compounding are accurately weighed, measured, or subdivided as appropriate to conform to the formula being prepared

Maintenance of Records
Every record required under this section must be:
- Kept by the pharmacy and be available, for at least two years for inspecting and copying by the board or its representative and to other authorized local, state, or federal law enforcement agencies
- Supplied by the pharmacy within 72 hours, if requested by an authorized agent of the Texas State Board of Pharmacy. If the pharmacy maintains the records in an electronic format, the requested records must be provided in an electronic format. Failure to provide the records set out in this section, either on site or within 72 hours, constitutes prima facie evidence of failure to keep and maintain records in violation of the Act

Compounding Records
- Compounding pursuant to patient specific prescription drug orders. Compounding records for all compounded preparations shall be maintained by the pharmacy electronically or manually as part of the prescription drug or medication order, formula record, formula book, or compounding log and shall include:
  - Date of preparation
  - Complete formula, including methodology and necessary equipment which includes the brand name(s) of the raw materials, or if no brand name, the generic name(s) or official name and

name(s) of the manufacturer(s) or distributor of the raw materials and the quantities of each
- o Signature or initials of the pharmacist or pharmacy technician or pharmacy technician trainee performing the compounding
- o Signature or initials of the pharmacist responsible for supervising pharmacy technicians or pharmacy technician trainees and conducting in-process and finals checks of compounded pharmaceuticals if pharmacy technicians or pharmacy technician trainees perform the compounding function
- o Quantity in units of finished preparation or amount of raw materials
- o Container used and the number of units prepared
- o Reference to the location of the following documentation which may be maintained with other records, such as quality control records:
    - Criteria used to determine the beyond-use date
    - Documentation of performance of quality control procedures
- Compounding records when batch compounding or compounding in anticipation of future prescription drug or medication orders
    - o Master work sheet. A master work sheet shall be developed and approved by a pharmacist for preparations prepared in batch. Once approved, a duplicate of the master work sheet shall be used as the preparation work sheet from which each batch is prepared and on which all documentation for that batch occurs. The master work sheet shall contain at a minimum:
        - Formula

- Components
- Compounding directions
- Sample label
- Evaluation and testing requirements
- Specific equipment used during preparation
- Storage requirements

o Preparation work sheet. The preparation work sheet for each batch of preparations shall document the following:

- Identity of all solutions and ingredients and their corresponding amounts, concentrations, or volumes
- Lot number for each component
- Component manufacturer/distributor or suitable identifying number
- Container specifications (e.g., syringe, pump cassette)
- Unique lot or control number assigned to batch
- Expiration date of batch-prepared preparation
- Date of preparation
- Name, initials, or electronic signature of the person(s) involved in the preparation
- Name, initials, or electronic signature of the responsible pharmacist
- Finished preparation evaluation and testing specifications, if applicable
- Comparison of actual yield to anticipated or theoretical yield, when appropriate

Office Use Compounding and Distribution of Sterile Compounded Preparations

- A pharmacy may compound, dispense, deliver, and distribute a compounded sterile preparation as specified in Subchapter D, Texas Pharmacy Act Chapter 562
- A Class A-S pharmacy is not required to register or be licensed under Chapter 431, Health and Safety Code, to distribute sterile compounded preparations to a Class C or Class C-S pharmacy
- A Class C-S pharmacy is not required to register or be licensed under Chapter 431, Health and Safety Code, to distribute sterile compounded preparations that the Class C-S pharmacy has compounded for other Class C or Class C-S pharmacies under common ownership
- To compound and deliver a compounded preparation under this subsection, a pharmacy must:
  - Verify the source of the raw materials to be used in a compounded drug
  - Comply with applicable United States Pharmacopoeia guidelines, including the testing requirements, and the Health Insurance Portability and Accountability Act of 1996
  - Enter into a written agreement with a practitioner for the practitioner's office use of a compounded preparation
  - Comply with all applicable competency and accrediting standards as determined by the board
- Written Agreement. A pharmacy that provides sterile compounded preparations to practitioners for office use or to another pharmacy shall enter into a written agreement with the practitioner or pharmacy. The written agreement shall:

- o Address acceptable standards of practice for a compounding pharmacy and a practitioner and receiving pharmacy that enter into the agreement including a statement that the compounded drugs may only be administered to the patient and may not be dispensed to the patient or sold to any other person or entity except to a veterinarian as authorized by §563.054 of the Act
  - o Require the practitioner or receiving pharmacy to include on a patient's chart, medication order or medication administration record the lot number and beyond-use date of a compounded preparation administered to a patient
  - o Describe the scope of services to be performed by the pharmacy and practitioner or receiving pharmacy, including a statement of the process for:
    - A patient to report an adverse reaction or submit a complaint; and
    - The pharmacy to recall batches of compounded preparations
- Records of orders and distribution of sterile compounded preparations to a practitioner for office use or to an institutional pharmacy for administration to a patient shall:
  - o Be kept by the pharmacy and be available, for at least two years from the date of the record, for inspecting and copying by the board or its representative and to other authorized local, state, or federal law enforcement agencies
  - o Maintained separately from the records of preparations dispensed pursuant to a prescription or medication order

- Supplied by the pharmacy within 72 hours, if requested by an authorized agent of the Texas State Board of Pharmacy or its representative. If the pharmacy maintains the records in an electronic format, the requested records must be provided in an electronic format. Failure to provide the records set out in this subsection, either on site or within 72 hours for whatever reason, constitutes prima facie evidence of failure to keep and maintain records
- Records may be maintained in an alternative data retention system, such as a data processing system or direct imaging system provided the data processing system is capable of producing a hard copy of the record upon the request of the board, its representative, or other authorized local, state, or federal law enforcement or regulatory agencies.
- Orders. The pharmacy shall maintain a record of all sterile compounded preparations ordered by a practitioner for office use or by an institutional pharmacy for administration to a patient. The record shall include the following information:
  - Date of the order
  - Name, address, and phone number of the practitioner who ordered the preparation and if applicable, the name, address and phone number of the institutional pharmacy ordering the preparation
  - Name, strength, and quantity of the preparation ordered.
- Distributions. The pharmacy shall maintain a record of all sterile compounded preparations distributed pursuant to an order to a practitioner for office use or by an institutional pharmacy for administration to a

patient. The record shall include the following information:

- o Date the preparation was compounded
- o Date the preparation was distributed
- o Name, strength and quantity in each container of the preparation
- o Pharmacy's lot number
- o Quantity of containers shipped
- o Name, address, and phone number of the practitioner or institutional pharmacy to whom the preparation is distributed

- The pharmacy shall store the order and distribution records of preparations for all sterile compounded preparations ordered by and or distributed to a practitioner for office use or by a pharmacy licensed to compound sterile preparations for administration to a patient in such a manner as to be able to provide an audit trail for all orders and distributions of any of the following during a specified time period:
  - o Any strength and dosage form of a preparation (by either brand or generic name or both)
  - o Any ingredient
  - o Any lot number
  - o Any practitioner
  - o Any facility
  - o Any pharmacy, if applicable

- The audit trail shall contain the following information:
  - o Date of order and date of the distribution
  - o Practitioner's name, address, and name of the institutional pharmacy, if applicable
  - o Name, strength and quantity of the preparation in each container of the preparation
  - o Name and quantity of each active ingredient
  - o Quantity of containers distributed
  - o Pharmacy's lot number

- Labeling. The pharmacy shall affix a label to the preparation containing the following information:
  - Name, address, and phone number of the compounding pharmacy
  - Statement: "For Institutional or Office Use Only-- Not for Resale"; or if the preparation is distributed to a veterinarian the statement: "Compounded Preparation"
  - Name and strength of the preparation or list of the active ingredients and strengths
  - Pharmacy's lot number
  - Beyond-use date as determined by the pharmacist using appropriate documented criteria
  - Quantity or amount in the container
  - Appropriate ancillary instructions, such as storage instructions or cautionary statements, including hazardous drug warning labels where appropriate
  - Device-specific instructions, where appropriate

Recall Procedures
- The pharmacy shall have written procedures for the recall of any compounded sterile preparation provided to a patient, to a practitioner for office use, or a pharmacy for administration. Written procedures shall include, but not be limited to the requirements as specified in this section
- The pharmacy shall immediately initiate a recall of any sterile preparation compounded by the pharmacy upon identification of a potential or confirmed harm to a patient
- In the event of a recall, the pharmacist-in-charge shall ensure that:

- Each practitioner, facility, and/or pharmacy to which the preparation was distributed is notified, in writing, of the recall
- Each patient to whom the preparation was dispensed is notified, in writing, of the recall
- The board is notified of the recall, in writing, not later than 24 hours after the recall is issued
- If the preparation is distributed for office use, the Texas Department of State Health Services, Drugs and Medical Devices Group, is notified of the recall, in writing
- The preparation is quarantined
- The pharmacy keeps a written record of the recall including all actions taken to notify all parties and steps taken to ensure corrective measures

- If a pharmacy fails to initiate a recall, the board may require a pharmacy to initiate a recall if there is potential for or confirmed harm to a patient
- A pharmacy that compounds sterile preparations shall notify the board immediately of any adverse effects reported to the pharmacy or that are known by the pharmacy to be potentially attributable to a sterile preparation compounded by the pharmacy

Section Thirty: Pseudoephederine Laws

Federal Laws

- Sold for personal use through face-to-face stores, mobile retail vendors, or through the mail
- Nonliquid (includes gelcaps) forms **must** be in unit dose packaging
- Report losses to the DEA (examples: theft, in-transit)
- Max of 3.6 grams per day per purchaser
- Max of 9 grams per 30-day period per purchaser
- Max of 7.5 grams per 30-day period per purchaser at a mobile retail vendor
- Customers may not have direct access to the products (e.g., store behind counter or in locked case)
- Seller must maintain a written (bound record book) or electronic list of each sale, including
  - Name of product
  - Quantity sold
  - Name of purchaser
  - Address of purchaser
  - Date and time of sale
  - Signature of purchaser
- Seller must keep the logbook for at least 2 years from the date of sale
- Each seller must do a self-certification with the DEA
- Sales personnel must be trained

Texas Laws

This chapter does not apply to the sale of any product dispensed or delivered by a pharmacist according to a prescription issued by a practitioner for a valid medical purpose and in the course of professional practice.

Who can sell?
- Business with a licensed pharmacy
- Business with no licensed pharmacy – must hold a certificate of authority

Where are the products located?
- In a business with a pharmacy – behind the pharmacy counter **or** in a locked case
  - Within 30 feet of pharmacy counter
  - In direct line of sight from a pharmacy counter
- In a business without a pharmacy – behind a sales counter **or** in a locked case
  - Within 30 feet of sales counter
  - In direct line of sight from a sales counter staffed continuously by an employee

Buying Procedure
- Requirements of the person making the purchase
  - Display a driver's license or other form of government-issued identification containing the person's photograph and indicating that the person is 16 years of age or older
  - Sign for the purchase
- Business must make a record of the sale
  - Name of the person making the purchase
  - Date of birth of the purchaser
  - Address of the purchaser

- o Type of identification supplied and identification number
- o Date and time of the purchase
- o Item and number of grams purchased

Maximum Amount
- Max of 3.6 grams per calendar day per purchaser
- Max of 9 grams within any 30-day period per purchaser

Transmission of Information
- Before completing an over-the-counter sale of a product containing ephedrine, pseudoephedrine, or norpseudoephedrine, a business establishment that engages in those sales shall transmit the information required to a real-time electronic logging system
- May not complete the sale if notified by the system that the maximum limits will be reached
- Override function available if the employee has a reasonable fear of imminent bodily injury or death from the person attempting to obtain the products
- If the system goes down then can maintain a written log and then enter the information into the real-time electronic logging system

Records
> Records must be kept for a minimum of 2 years

Products Affected
> Does not apply to the liquid, liquid capsule, or liquid gel capsule form

Section Thirty-One: Therapeutic Optometrists

- Optometrist – may not prescribe
- Therapeutic optometrist – may prescribe certain topical medications for the purpose of diagnosing and treating visual defects, abnormal conditions, and diseases of the human vision system
- Optometric Glaucoma Specialist – may prescribe anything a Therapeutic Optometrist can and may prescribe the following oral medications:
  - One 10-day supply of antibiotics
  - One 72-hour supply of antihistamines
  - One 7-day supply of non-steroidal anti-inflammatories
  - One 3-day supply of any analgesic in Schedule III, IV, and V
  - Antiglaucoma drugs

Prescriptions by a Therapeutic Optometrist

- To prohibit substitution of a generically equivalent drug product on a written prescription drug order, a therapeutic optometrist must write across the face of the written prescription, in the therapeutic optometrist's own handwriting, "brand necessary" or "brand medically necessary." If the therapeutic optometrist does not clearly indicate "brand necessary" or "brand medically necessary," the pharmacist may substitute a generically equivalent drug product
- All prescriptions shall contain the following information:
  - The date of issuance

- Name and address of the patient for whom the drug is prescribed
- Name, strength, and quantity of the drug, medicine, or device prescribed
- Direction for use of the drug, medicine, or device prescribed
- Name and address of the therapeutic optometrist
- Manually written signature of the prescribing therapeutic optometrist; or an electronic signature provided that the prescription is electronically signed by the practitioner using a system which electronically replicates the practitioner's manual signature on the written prescription, and provided:
  - That security features of the system require the practitioner to authorize each use; and
  - Prescription is printed on paper that is designed to prevent unauthorized copying of a completed prescription and to prevent the erasure or modification of information written on the prescription by the prescribing practitioner; and
- License number of the prescribing therapeutic optometrist including the therapeutic designation
- The prescribing therapeutic optometrist issuing verbal or electronic prescription drug orders to a pharmacist shall furnish the same information required for a written prescription, except for the written signature. If the therapeutic optometrist does not clearly indicate "brand necessary" or "brand medically necessary," when communicating the prescription to the pharmacist, the pharmacist may substitute a generically equivalent drug

- A therapeutic optometrist may charge a reasonable fee for drugs administered within the optometric office, but a therapeutic optometrist shall not charge for any drugs supplied to the patient as take-home medication. Any drug supplied by a therapeutic optometrist other than an over-the counter drug shall be labeled in compliance with the following information in compliance with the Texas Dangerous Drug Act shall contain the following:
    - Name, address and telephone number of the therapeutic optometrist
    - Date of dispensing
    - Name of the patient
    - Name and strength of the drug
    - Directions for use
- At least annually, the Texas Optometry Board shall provide to the Texas State Board of Pharmacy a list of the topical ocular pharmaceutical agents which may be prescribed by therapeutic optometrist
- A therapeutic optometrist may administer and prescribe all:
    - Ophthalmic devices
    - Over-the-counter oral medications; and
    - Appropriate topical pharmaceutical agents used for diagnosing and treating visual defects, abnormal conditions, and diseases of the human eye and adnexa, which are included in the following classifications or are combinations of agents in the classifications. No drug falling within one of the following categories may be used for the treatment of glaucoma in a manner that was not permitted by law on August 31, 1991:
        - Anti-allergy:
            - Antihistamine
            - Membrane stabilizer

- Anti-fungal:
  - Imidazoles
  - Polyenes
- Anti-infective:
  - Aminoglycoside
  - Anti-cell membrane
  - Anti-cell wall synthesis
  - Anti-DNA synthesis
  - Anti-protein synthesis (excluding chloramphenicol)
  - Anti-ACHase
  - Cephalosporin
  - Agents affecting intermediary metabolism
- Anti-inflammatory:
  - Nonsteroidal anti-inflammatory drug (NSAID)
  - Steroid
- Antiseptic
- Chelating agent
- Chemical cautery
- Cycloplegic: parasympatholytic
- Hyperosmotic
- Miotic:
  - Anti-ACHase
  - Parasympathomimetic
- Mucolytic
- Mydriatic: sympathomimetic (Alpha 1 agonists only)
- Vasoconstrictor: sympathomimetic (Alpha 1 agonists only)
- Antivirals

- A therapeutic optometrist may possess and administer cocaine eye drops for diagnostic purpose. The cocaine eye drops must be no greater than 10 percent solution in prepackaged liquid form
    - A therapeutic optometrist must observe all requirements of the Texas Controlled Substances Act, the Health and Safety Code, Chapter 481, and all requirements of the Texas Department of Public Safety (DPS) Drug Rules, in making application and maintaining renewal of a United States Drug Enforcement Administration (DEA) registration number for possession of the cocaine eye drops, a Schedule II controlled substance
    - A therapeutic optometrist must obtain a registration number from the DPS for the principal office of practice. Application may be made for a separate registration for the practice of optometry at a satellite office but all requirements of this rule shall apply in all locations
    - The therapeutic optometrist must use the required DEA form for the purchase of the cocaine eye drops and shall maintain a complete and accurate record of purchases (to include samples received from pharmaceutical manufacturer representatives) and administration of controlled substances. The maximum amount to be purchased and maintained in an office of practice shall be no more than two vials, one opened and one in inventory
    - The recordkeeping listed in this section shall be subject to inspection at all times by the Texas Department of Public Safety, the U.S. Drug

Enforcement Administration, and the Texas Optometry Board and any officer or employee of the governmental agencies shall have the right to inspect and copy records, reports, and other documents, and inspect security controls, inventory and premises where such cocaine eye drops are possessed or administered
- Minimum security controls shall be established to include but not limited to:
  - Establishing adequate security to prevent unauthorized access and diversion of the controlled substance
  - During the course of business activities, not allowing any individual access to the storage area for controlled substances except those authorized by the therapeutic optometrist
  - Storing the controlled substance in a securely locked, substantially constructed cabinet or security cabinet which shall meet the requirements under the DPS Drug Rules
  - Not employ in any manner an individual that would have access to controlled substances who has had a federal or state application for controlled substances denied or revoked, or have been convicted of a felony offense under any state or federal law relating to controlled substances or been convicted of any other felony, or have been a licensee of a health regulatory agency whose license has been revoked, canceled, or suspended

Definitions

Accurately as prescribed – distributing and/or delivering a medication drug order:
- To the correct patient (or agent of the patient) for whom the drug or device was prescribed
- With the correct drug in the correct strength, quantity, and dosage form ordered by the practitioner; **and**
- With correct labeling as ordered by the practitioner and required by rule

Administer – to directly apply a prescription drug to the body of a patient by any means—including injection, inhalation, or ingestion—by a person authorized by law to administer the drug, including a practitioner, an authorized agent under a practitioner's supervision, or the patient at the direction of a practitioner

Adultered –
- Contains any filthy substance
- Prepared/packaged/stored where it may have been contaminated
- Good manufacturing practices not followed
- Container may contaminate the drug
- Unsafe color additive
- Strength differs (95-105% is ok) from what listed on the label

335

- Misfilled – drug has been substituted

Airborne particulate cleanliness class – the level of cleanliness specified by the maximum allowable number of particles per cubic meter of air as specified in the International Organization of Standardization (ISO) Classification Air Cleanliness. For example:
- ISO Class 5 is an atmospheric environment that contains fewer than 3,520 particles 0.5 microns in diameter per cubic meter of air (formerly stated as 100 particles 0.5 microns in diameter per cubic foot of air)
- ISO Class 7 is an atmospheric environment that contains fewer than 352,000 particles 0.5 microns in diameter per cubic meter of air (formerly stated as 10,000 particles 0.5 microns in diameter per cubic foot of air)
- ISO Class 8 is an atmospheric environment that contains fewer than 3,520,000 particles 0.5 microns in diameter per cubic meter of air (formerly stated as 100,000 particles 0.5 microns in diameter per cubic foot of air)

Ambulatory surgical center (ASC) – a freestanding facility that is licensed by the Texas Department of State Health Services to provide surgical services to patients who do not require overnight hospital care

Ancillary supplies – supplies necessary for the preparation and administration of compounded sterile preparations

Anteroom – an ISO Class 8 or better area where personnel may perform hand hygiene and garbing procedures, staging of components, order entry, labeling, and other high-particulate generating activities. It is also a transition area that:

- Provides assurance that pressure relationships are constantly maintained so that air flows from clean to dirty areas; **and**
- Reduces the need for the heating, ventilating and air conditioning (HVAC) control system to respond to large disturbances

Approved provider – an individual, institution, organization, association, corporation, or agency that is approved by the board

Aseptic Processing – the technique involving procedures designed to preclude contamination of drugs, packaging, equipment, or supplies by microorganisms during preparation

Automated checking device – a device that confirms that the correct drug and strength has been labeled with the correct label for the correct patient prior to delivery of the drug to the patient

Automated compounding or counting device – an automated device that compounds, measures, counts, and/or packages a specified quantity of dosage units of a designated drug product

Automated drug dispensing system – an automated device that measures, counts, and/or packages a specified quantity of dosage units for a designated drug product

Automated medication supply system – a mechanical system that performs operations or activities relative to the storage and distribution of medications for administration and which collects, controls, and maintains all transaction information

Automated pharmacy system – a mechanical system that dispenses prescription drugs and maintains related transaction information.

Batch – a specific quantity of a drug or other material that is intended to have uniform character and quality, within specified limits, and is produced during a single preparation cycle

Batch preparation compounding – compounding of multiple sterile preparation units, in a single discrete process, by the same individual(s), carried out during one (1) limited time period. Batch preparation/compounding does not include the preparation of multiple sterile preparation units pursuant to patient specific medication orders

Beyond-use date – the date or time after which the compounded preparation shall not be stored or transported or begin to be administered to a patient. The beyond-use date is determined from the date or time the preparation is compounded

Biological safety cabinet, Class II – a ventilated cabinet for personnel, product, and environmental protection, having an open front with inward airflow for personnel protection, downward HEPA filtered laminar airflow for product protection, and HEPA filtered exhausted air for environmental protection.

Board – the Texas State Board of Pharmacy

Buffer area, buffer or core Room, buffer or clean room areas, buffer room area, buffer or clean area, or buffer zone – an ISO Class 7 area where the primary engineering control area is physically located. Activities that occur in this area include the preparation and staging of components and supplies used when compounding sterile preparations

Centralized prescription dispensing – the dispensing or refilling of a prescription drug order by a Class A (community), Class C (institutional), or Class E (non-resident) pharmacy at the request of another Class A (community), or Class C (institutional), and the return of the dispensed prescriptions to the requesting pharmacy for delivery to the patient or patient's agent or, at the request of the requesting pharmacy, direct delivery to the patient

Certificate of completion – a certificate or other official document presented to a participant upon the successful completion of an approved continuing education program

Class A pharmacy license – community pharmacy

Class B pharmacy license – nuclear pharmacy

Class C pharmacy license – institutional pharmacy

Class D pharmacy license – clinic pharmacy

Class E pharmacy license – non-resident pharmacy, a pharmacy located in another state whose primary business is to:
- Dispense a prescription drug or device under a prescription drug order and
- To deliver the drug or device to the patient, including a patient in this state, by the United States mail, common carrier, or delivery service

Class F pharmacy license – pharmacy located in a freestanding emergency medical care center

Class G pharmacy license – central prescription drug or medication order processing pharmacy

Class H pharmacy license – limited prescription delivery pharmacy

Clean room or controlled area – a room in which the concentration of airborne particles is controlled to meet a specified airborne particulate cleanliness class. Microorganisms in the environment are monitored so that a microbial level for air, surface, and personnel gear are not exceeded for a specified cleanliness class

Clinic – a facility/location other than a physician's office, where limited types of dangerous drugs or devices restricted to those listed in and approved for the clinic's formulary are stored, administered, provided, or dispensed to outpatients

Clinical pharmacy program – an ongoing program in which pharmacists are on-duty during the time the pharmacy is open for pharmacy services, and pharmacists provide direct, focused, medication-related care for the purpose of optimizing patients' medication therapy and achieving definite outcomes, which includes the following activities:
- Prospective medication therapy consultation, selection, and adjustment
- Monitoring laboratory values and therapeutic drug monitoring

- Identifying and resolving medication-related problems; and
- Disease state management

College/School of pharmacy – a college/school of pharmacy whose professional degree progam has been accredited by ACPE and approved by the board

Component – any ingredient intended for use in the compounding of a drug preparation, including those that may not appear in such preparation

Compounding – means the preparation, mixing, assembling, packaging, or labeling of a drug or device
- As the result of a practitioner's prescription drug order based on the practitioner-patient-pharmacist relationship in the course of professional practice
- For administration to a patient by a practitioner as the result of a practitioner's initiative based on the practitioner-patient-pharmacist relationship in the course of professional practice
- In anticipation of a prescription drug order based on a routine, regularly observed prescribing pattern
- For or as an incident to research, teaching, or chemical analysis and not for selling or dispensing

Compounding aseptic isolator – a form of barrier isolator specifically designed for compounding pharmaceutical ingredients or preparations. It is designed to maintain an aseptic compounding environment within the isolator throughout the compounding and material transfer processes. Air exchange into the isolator from the surrounding environment shall not occur unless it has first passed through a microbial retentive filter (HEPA minimum)

Compounding aseptic containment isolator – a compounding aseptic isolator designed to provide worker protection from exposure to undesirable levels of airborne drug throughout the compounding and material transfer processes and to provide an aseptic environment for compounding sterile preparations. Air exchange with the surrounding environment should not occur unless the air is first passed through a microbial retentive filter (HEPA minimum) system capable of containing airborne concentrations of the physical size and state of the drug being compounded. Where volatile hazardous drugs are prepared, the exhaust air from the isolator should be appropriately removed by properly designed building ventilation

Confidential record – any health-related record containing information that identifies an individual and that is maintained by a pharmacy or pharmacist, like a patient medication record, prescription drug order, or medication drug order

Consultant pharmacist – a pharmacist retained by a facility on a routine basis to consult with the facility in areas that pertain to the practice of pharmacy

Continuous supervision – supervision provided by the pharmacist-in-charge, consultant pharmacist, and/or staff pharmacist, and consists of on-site and telephone supervision, routine inspection, and a policy and procedure manual

Controlled substance - a substance, including a drug, listed in Schedule I, II, III, IV, or V

CPE Monitor – a collaborative service from the National Association of Boards of Pharmacy and ACPE that provides an electronic system for pharmacists to track their completed CPE credits

Critical area – a critical area is an ISO Class 5 environment

Critical sites – sterile ingredients of compounded sterile preparations and locations on devices and components used to prepare, package, and transfer compounded sterile preparations that provide opportunity for exposure to contamination

Cytotoxic – a pharmaceutical that has the capability of killing living cells

Dangerous drug – a device or a drug that is unsafe for self-medication and that is not included in Schedules I through V. The term includes a device or a drug that bears or is required to bear the legend:

- Caution: Federal law prohibits dispensing without prescription" or "Rx only" or another legend that complies with federal law; **or**
- "Caution: Federal law restricts this drug to use by or on the order of a licensed veterinarian."

Deceit – the assertion, as a fact, of that which is not true, for the purpose of deceiving or defrauding another

Deliver – to sell, dispense, give away, or supply in any other manner

Device – an instrument, apparatus, implement, machine, contrivance, implant, *in vitro* reagent, or other similar or related article, including a component part or accessory, that is required under federal or state law to be ordered or prescribed by a practitioner

Designated agent – an individual, including a licensed nurse, physician assistant, or pharmacist

- Who is designated by a practitioner and authorized to communicate a prescription drug order to a pharmacist **and**
- For whom the practitioner assumes legal responsibility

Direct compounding area – a critical area within the ISO Class 5 primary engineering control where critical sites are exposed to unidirectional HEPA-filtered air, also known as first air

Direct copy – electronic copy or carbonized copy of a medication order, including a facsimile (FAX) or digital image

Disinfectant – a disinfectant is an agent that frees from infection, usually a chemical agent but sometimes a physical one, and that destroys disease-causing pathogens or other harmful microorganisms but may not kill bacterial spores. It refers to substances applied to inanimate objects

Dispense – to prepare, package, compound, or label a dangerous drug in the course of professional practice for delivery under the lawful order of a practitioner to an ultimate user or the user's agent

Dispensing error – an action committed by a pharmacist or other pharmacy personnel that causes the patient or patient's agent to take possession of a dispensed prescription drug and in individual subsequently discovers that the patient has received an incorrect drug product, which includes incorrect strength, incorrect dosage form, and/or incorrect directions for use

Distribute – to deliver a prescription drug or device other than by administering or dispensing.

Distributing pharmacist – the pharmacist who checks the medication order prior to distribution

Downtime – period of time during which a data processing system is not operable

Drug –
- Substance recognized as a drug in a drug compendium, including the current official United States Pharmacopoeia, official National Formulary, or official Homeopathic Pharmacopoeia, or in a supplement to a drug compendium
- Substance intended for use in the diagnosis, cure, mitigation, treatment, or prevention of disease in a human or another animal
- Substance, other than food, intended to affect the structure or a function of the body of a human or another animal
- Dangerous drug
- Controlled substance

Drug regimen review – evaluation of prescription drug or medication orders and a patient medication record for
- Known allergy
- Rational therapy-contraindication

- Reasonable dose and route of administration
- Reasonable directions for use
- Duplication of therapy
- Drug-drug interaction
- Drug-food interaction
- Drug-disease interaction
- Adverse drug reaction
- Proper use, including overuse or underuse.

Electronic signature – a unique security code or other identifier that specifically identifies the person entering information into a data processing system. A facility which utilizes electronic signatures must:
- Maintain a permanent list of the unique security codes assigned to persons authorized to use the data processing system; **and**
- Have an ongoing security program which is capable of identifying misuse and/or unauthorized use of electronic signatures

Emergency medication kits – controlled substances and dangerous drugs maintained by a provider pharmacy to meet the emergency medication needs of a resident:
- At an institution licensed under Chapter 242 or 252, Health and Safety Code; **or**
- At an institution licensed under Chapter 242, Health and Safety Code and that is a veterans home as defined by the §164.002, Natural Resources Code, if the

provider pharmacy is a United States Department of Veterans Affairs pharmacy or another federally operated pharmacy

Expiration date – the date (and time, when applicable) beyond which a product should not be used

Extended-intern – registered intern who has done one of the following:
- Applied for licensure by examination, passed NAPLEX® and Texas MPJE®, but not enough internship hours
- Applied to take the NAPLEX and Texas Jurisprudence Examinations within six (6) calendar months after graduation and has either:
  - Has graduated and received diploma; **or**
  - Ready to graduate (completed all of the requirements for graduation)
- Applied to take the NAPLEX® and Texas Jurisprudence Examinations within six (6) calendar months after obtaining full certification from the Foreign Pharmacy Graduate Equivalency Commission
- Applied to the Board for re-issuance of a pharmacist license which has been expired for more than 2 years but fewer than 10 years and has successfully passed the Texas Pharmacy Jurisprudence examination, but lacks the required number of hours of internship or continuing education required for licensure
- Been ordered by the Board to complete an internship

Facility –
- Hospital or other patient facility that is licensed under Chapter 241 or 577, Health and Safety Code
- Hospice patient facility that is licensed under Chapter 142, Health and Safety Code
- Ambulatory surgical center licensed under Chapter 243, Health and Safety Code; **or**
- Hospital maintained or operated by the state

First air – the air exiting the HEPA filter in a unidirectional air stream that is essentially particle-free

Floor stock – prescription drugs or devices not labeled for a specific patient and maintained at a nursing station or other hospital department (excluding the pharmacy) for the purpose of administration to a patient of the facility

Foreign pharmacy graduate – a pharmacist whose pharmacy degree was conferred by a pharmacy school whose professional degree program has not been accredited by ACPE and approved by the board

Formulary – list of drugs approved for use in the facility by the committee which performs the pharmacy and therapeutics function for the facility

Fraud – an intentional perversion of truth for the purpose of inducing another to part with some valuable thing belonging to him, to surrender a legal right, or to issue a license; a false representation of a matter of fact, whether by words or by conduct, by false or misleading allegations, or by concealment of that which should have been disclosed, which deceives or is intended to deceive another

Full-time pharmacist – a pharmacist who works in a pharmacy from 30 to 40 hours per week—or, if the pharmacy, is open fewer than 60 hours per week, one-half of the time the pharmacy is open

Generically equivalent – both pharmaceutically and therapeutically equivalent

Gross immorality – shall include, but not be limited to:
- Conduct which is willful, flagrant, and shameless, and which shows a moral indifference to standards of the community
- Engaging in an act which is a felony
- Engaging in an act that constitutes sexually deviant behavior; **or**
- Being required to register with the Department of Public Safety as a sex offender

Hard copy – a physical document that is readable without the use of a special device (e.g., data processing system or computer)

Hot water – the temperature of water from the pharmacy's sink, maintained at a minimum of 105 degrees F (41 degrees C)

HVAC – heating, ventilation, and air conditioning

Immediate use – a sterile preparation that is not prepared according to USP 797 standards (e.g. outside the pharmacy and most likely not by pharmacy personnel), which shall be stored for no longer than one (1) hour after completion of the preparation

Indigent – person who meets or falls below 185% of federal poverty income guidelines as established from time to time by the United States Department of Health and Human Services

Institutional pharmacy – area or areas in a facility where drugs are stored, bulk compounded, delivered, compounded, dispensed, and distributed to other areas or departments of the facility, or dispensed to an ultimate user or his or her agent

Intern-trainee – a pharmacist intern, registered with the board, who is enrolled in the first year of the professional sequence of a Texas college/school of pharmacy and who may only work during times and in sites assigned by a Texas college/school of pharmacy

Internship – a practical experience program that is approved by the board

Initial license period – the time period between the date of issuance of a pharmacist's license and the next expiration date following the initial 30 day expiration date

Investigational new drug – new drug intended for investigational use by experts qualified to evaluate the safety and effectiveness of the drug as authorized by the Food and Drug Administration

Label – written, printed, or graphic matter on the immediate container of a drug or device

Labeling – the process of affixing a label, including all information required by federal and state statute or regulation, to a drug or device container. The term does **not** include:
- Labeling by a manufacturer, packer, or distributor of a nonprescription drug or commercially packaged prescription drug or device
- Unit dose packaging

Limited type of device – an instrument, apparatus, implement, machine, contrivance, implant, in vitro reagent, or other similar or related article, including any component part or accessory, that is required under federal or state law to be ordered or prescribed by a practitioner, that is contained in the clinic formulary and is to be administered, dispensed, or provided according to the objectives of the clinic.

Limited type of drug – a dangerous drug contained in the clinic formulary, and to be administered, dispensed, or provided according to the objectives of the clinic.

Live programs – activities that provide for direct interaction between faculty and participants and may include lectures, symposia, live teleconferences, workshops, etc

Manufacturer – a person, other than a pharmacist, who manufactures dangerous drugs. The term includes a person who prepares dangerous drugs in dosage form by mixing, compounding, encapsulating, entableting, or any other process

Manufacturing – the production, preparation, propagation, conversion, or processing of a drug or device, either directly or indirectly, by extraction from a substance of natural origin or independently by a chemical or biological synthesis. The term includes packaging or repackaging a substance or labeling or relabeling a container and promoting and marketing the drug or device and preparing and promoting a commercially available product from a bulk compound for resale by a person, including a pharmacy or practitioner. The term does not include compounding

Media-fill test – a media-fill test is used to qualify aseptic technique of compounding personnel or processes and to ensure that the processes used are able to produce sterile preparation without microbial contamination

Medication order – an order from a practitioner or a practitioner's designated agent for administration of a drug or device

Midlevel practitioner – advanced practice nurse, physician assistant

Misbranded –
- Labeling is false or misleading
- Labeling fails to meet manufacturer's labeling requirements
  - Name and address of manufacturer
  - Quantity
  - Generic and brand name of drug if applicable
  - Strength of the drug
  - Information for use
  - Warnings against use
  - Expiration date
- Pharmacist fills a prescription without authorization from prescriber

- Counterfeit drug
- Packaging violates Poison Prevention Packaging Act

Misrepresentation – a manifestation by words or other conduct which is a false representation of a matter of fact

Multiple-dose container – a multiple-unit container for articles or preparations intended for potential administration only and usually contains antimicrobial preservatives. The beyond-use date for an opened or entered (e.g., needle-punctured) multiple-dose container with antimicrobial preservatives is 28 days, unless otherwise specified by the manufacturer.

Narcotic – contains opium or an opiate derivative

Negative pressure room – a room that is at a lower pressure compared to adjacent spaces and, therefore, the net flow of air is into the room

New prescription drug order – a prescription drug order that:
- Has not been dispensed to the patient in the same strength and dosage form by this pharmacy within the past year
- Is transferred from another pharmacy and/or
- Is a discharge prescription drug order. (Note: furlough prescription drug orders are not considered new prescription drug orders)

Nonprescription drug – a nonnarcotic drug or device that may be sold without a prescription and that is labeled and packaged in compliance with state or federal law

Office use – the administration of a compounded drug to a patient by a practitioner in the practitioner's office or by the practitioner in a health care facility or treatment setting, including a hospital, ambulatory surgical center, or for administration or provision by a veterinarian

Outpatient – an ambulatory patient who comes to a clinic to receive services related to the objectives of the clinic and departs the same day

Over-the-counter (OTC) – safe and effective for self-use with properly labeled directions

Part-time pharmacist – a pharmacist either employed or under contract, who routinely works less than full-time

Patient –
- an individual for whom a dangerous drug is prescribed or to whom a dangerous drug is administered; **or**
- an owner or the agent of an owner of an animal for which a dangerous drug is prescribed or to which a dangerous drug is administered

Patient counseling – communication by a pharmacist of information, as specified by board rule, to a patient or caregiver to improve therapy by ensuring proper use of a drug or device

Patient med-pak – a package prepared by a pharmacist for a specific patient comprised of a series of containers and containing two or more prescribed solid oral dosage forms. The patient med-pak is so designed or each container is labeled as to indicate the day and time or period of time that the contents within each container are to be taken

Perpetual inventory – an inventory which documents all receipts and distributions of a drug product, such that an accurate, current balance of the amount of the drug product present in the pharmacy is indicated

Person – an individual, corporation, partnership, and association

Pharmaceutical care – providing drug therapy and other pharmaceutical services defined by board rule and intended to assist in curing or preventing a disease, eliminating or reducing a patient's symptom, or arresting or slowing a disease process

Pharmaceutically equivalent – identical amounts of the same active chemical ingredients in the same dosage form

358

Pharmacist – a person licensed by the Texas State Board of Pharmacy to practice pharmacy

Pharmacist-in-charge (PIC) – the pharmacist designated on a pharmacy license as the pharmacist who has the authority or responsibility for the pharmacy's compliance with statutes and rules relating to the practice of pharmacy

Pharmacist-intern – an intern-trainee, a student-intern, or an extended-intern who is participating in a board approved internship program

Pharmacist preceptor – a pharmacist licensed in Texas to practice pharmacy who meets the requirements under board rules and is recognized by the board to supervise and be responsible for the activities and functions of a pharmacist-intern in an internship program

Pharmacy – a facility where prescription drug or medication orders are received, processed, dispensed, or distributed

Pharmacy and therapeutics function – committee of the medical staff in the facility which assists in the formulation of broad professional policies regarding the evaluation, selection, distribution, handling, use, and administration, and all other matters relating to the use of drugs and devices in the facility

Pharmacy bulk package – a container of a sterile preparation for potential use that contains many single doses. The contents are intended for use in a pharmacy admixture program and are restricted to the preparation of admixtures for infusion or, through a sterile transfer device, for the filling of empty sterile syringes. The closure shall be penetrated only one (1) time after constitution with a suitable sterile transfer device or dispensing set, which allows measured dispensing of the contents. The pharmacy bulk package is to be used only in a suitable work area such as a laminar flow hood (or an equivalent clean air compounding area)

Pharmacy technician – an individual employed by a pharmacy whose responsibility is to provide technical services that do not require professional judgment regarding preparing and distributing drugs and who works under the direct supervision of and is responsible to a pharmacist

Pharmacy technician trainee – an individual who is registered with the board as a pharmacy technician trainee and is authorized to participate in a pharmacy's technician training program

Practice of pharmacy –
- Provision of those acts or services necessary to provide pharmaceutical care
- Interpretation and evaluation of prescription drug orders or medication orders

360

- Participation in drug and device selection as authorized by law, drug administration, drug regimen review, or drug or drug-related research
- Provision of patient counseling
- Responsibility for
    - Dispensing of prescription drug orders or distribution of medication orders in the patient's best interest
    - Compounding and labeling of drugs and devices, except labeling by a manufacturer, repackager, or distributor of nonprescription drugs and commercially packaged prescription drugs and devices
    - Proper and safe storage of drugs and devices
    - Maintenance of proper records for drugs and devices
- Performance of a specific act of drug therapy management for a patient delegated to a pharmacist by a written protocol from a physician

Practitioner – a person licensed
- By the Texas State Board of Medical Examiners, State Board of Dental Examiners, Texas State Board of Podiatric Medical Examiners, Texas Optometry Board, or State Board of Veterinary Medical Examiners to prescribe and administer dangerous drugs

- By another state in a health field in which, under the laws of Texas, a licensee may legally prescribe dangerous drugs
- In Canada or Mexico in a health field in which, under the laws of Texas, a licensee may legally prescribe dangerous drugs
- An advanced practice nurse or physician assistant to whom a physician has delegated the authority to carry out or sign prescription drug orders

Prepackaging – the act of repackaging and re-labeling quantities of drug products from a manufacturer's original container into unit-dose packaging or a multiple dose container for distribution within the facility

Prepackaging (in regards to emergency medication kits) – the act of repackaging and relabeling quantities of drug products from a manufacturer's original commercial container, or quantities of unit dosed drugs, into another cartridge or container for dispensing by a pharmacist using an emergency medication kit.

Preparation or compounded sterile preparation – a sterile admixture compounded in a licensed pharmacy or other healthcare-related facility pursuant to the order of a licensed prescriber

Prescription – an order from a practitioner, or an agent of the practitioner designated in writing as authorized to communicate prescriptions to a pharmacist for a dangerous drug to be dispensed that states

- Date of the order's issue
- Name and address of the patient
    - If the drug is prescribed for an animal, the species of the animal
- Name and quantity of the drug prescribed
- Directions for the use of the drug
- Intended use of the drug, unless the practitioner determines the furnishing of this information is not in the best interest of the patient
- Name, address, and telephone number of the practitioner at the practitioner's usual place of business, legibly printed or stamped
- Name, address, and telephone number of the licensed midwife, registered nurse, or physician assistant, legibly printed or stamped (if signed by a licensed midwife, registered nurse, or physician assistant)

Prescription drug –

- Substance for which federal or state law requires a prescription before the substance may be legally dispensed to the public
- Drug or device that under federal law is required, before being dispensed or delivered, to be labeled with the statement

- o "Caution: Federal law prohibits dispensing without prescription" or "Rx only" or another legend that complies with federal law
- o "Caution: Federal law restricts this drug to use by or on the order of a licensed veterinarian"
- Drug or device that is required by federal or state statute or regulation to be dispensed on prescription or that is restricted to use by a practitioner only
- Habit-forming, toxic or potential for harm or the use requires physician supervision

Prescription drug order – an order from a practitioner or a practitioner's designated agent to a pharmacist for a drug or device to be dispensed

Primary engineering control – a device or room that provides an ISO Class 5 environment for the exposure of critical sites when compounding sterile preparations. Such devices include but may not be limited to: laminar airflow workbenches, biological safety cabinets, and compounding aseptic isolators and compounding aseptic containment isolators

Positive control – quality assurance sample prepared to test positive for microbial growth

Positive pressure room – a room that is at a higher pressure compared to adjacent spaces, and therefore, the net airflow goes out of the room

Probation – the suspension of a sanction imposed against a license during good behavior, for a term and under conditions as determined by the board

Product – a product is a commercially manufactured sterile drug or nutrient that has been evaluated for safety and efficacy by the U.S. Food and Drug Administration (FDA). Products are accompanied by full prescribing information, which is commonly known as the FDA-approved manufacturer's labeling or product package insert

Prospective drug use review – the review of a patient's drug therapy and prescription drug order or medication order, as defined by board rule, before dispensing or distributing a drug to the patient

Provide – to supply one or more unit doses of a nonprescription drug or dangerous drug to a patient.

Provider pharmacy – the community pharmacy (Class A) or the institutional pharmacy (Class C) providing remote pharmacy services

Provider pharmacy (in regards to emergency medication kits)– the community pharmacy (Class A); the institutional pharmacy (Class C); the non-resident (Class E) pharmacy located not more than 20 miles from an institution licensed under Chapter 242 or 252, Health and Safety Code; or the United States Department of Veterans Affairs pharmacy or another federally operated pharmacy providing remote pharmacy services

Quality assurance – the set of activities used to ensure that the process used in the preparation of sterile drug preparations lead to preparations that meet predetermined standards of quality

Quality control – the set of testing activities used to determine that the ingredients, components (e.g., containers), and final compounded sterile preparations prepared meet predetermined requirements with respect to identity, purity, non-pyrogenicity, and sterility

Radioactive drug – a drug that exhibits spontaneous disintegration of unstable nuclei with the emission of nuclear particles or photons, including a nonradioactive reagent kit or nuclide generator that is intended to be used in the preparation of the substance

Readily retrievable – means that records shall be asterisked, redlined, or in some other manner readily identifiable apart from all other items appearing on the record

Real-time electronic logging system – means a system intended to be used by law enforcement agencies and pharmacies or other business establishments that:
- Is installed, operated, and maintained free of any one-time or recurring charge to the business establishment or to the state
- Is able to communicate in real time with similar systems operated in other states and similar systems containing information submitted by more than one state
- Complies with the security policy of the Criminal Justice Information Services division of the Federal Bureau of Investigation
- Complies with information exchange standards adopted by the National Information Exchange Model
- Uses a mechanism to prevent the completion of a sale of a product containing ephedrine, pseudoephedrine, or norpseudoephedrine that would violate state or federal law regarding the purchase of a product containing those substances; and
- Is equipped with an override of the mechanism that:
  - May be activated by an employee of a business establishment; and
  - Creates a record of each activation of the override

367

Reasonable quantity – an amount of a compounded drug that:

- Does not exceed the amount a practitioner anticipates may be used in the practitioner's office or facility before the beyond-use date of the drug
- Is reasonable considering the intended use of the compounded drug and the nature of the practitioner's practice; and
- For any practitioner and all practitioners as a whole, is not greater than the amount the pharmacy is capable of compounding in compliance with pharmaceutical standards for identity, strength, quality, and purity of the compounded drug, consistent with United States Pharmacopoeia guidelines and accreditation practices

Record – a notification, order form, statement, invoice, prescription, inventory information, or other document for the acquisition or disposal of a controlled substance

Remote pharmacy service – the provision of pharmacy services, including the storage and dispensing of prescription drugs, in remote sites

Remote site – a facility not located at the same location as a Class A or Class C pharmacy, at which remote pharmacy services are provided using an automated pharmacy dispensing system

Remote site (in regards to emergency medication kits) – a facility not located at the same location as a Class A, Class C, or Class E pharmacy or a United States Department of Affairs pharmacy or another federally operated pharmacy, at which remote pharmacy services are provided using an emergency medication kit

Reprimand – a public and formal censure against a license

Resident intern – an individual who:
- Has graduated from a college/school of pharmacy; and
- Is completing a residency program in the state of Texas accredited by the American Society of Health-System Pharmacists

Restrict – to limit, confine, abridge, narrow, or restrain a license for a term and under conditions determined by the board

Retire – a license has been withdrawn and is of no further force and effect

Revoke – a license is void and may not be reissued; however, upon the expiration of 12 months from and after the effective date of the order revoking a pharmacist license, application may be made to the board by the former licensee for the issuance of a license upon the successful completion of any examination required by the board

Rural hospital – a licensed hospital with 75 beds or fewer that:

- Located in a county with a population of 50,000 or less as defined by the United States Census Bureau in the most recent U.S. census; **or**
- Has been designated by the Centers for Medicare and Medicaid Services as a critical access hospital, rural referral center, or sole community hospital

Sample – a prescription drug that is not intended to be sold and is intended to promote the sale of the drug

Segregated compounding area – a designated space, either a demarcated area or room, that is restricted to preparing low-risk level compounded sterile preparations with 12-hour or less beyond-use date. Such area shall contain a device that provides unidirectional airflow of ISO Class 5 air quality for preparation of compounded sterile preparations and shall be void of activities and materials that are extraneous to sterile compounding

Single-dose container – a container intended for a single use, other than single-dose vials and single-dose large volume potential solutions. Examples of single-dose containers include pre-filled syringes, cartridges, and fusion-sealed containers without preservatives

Single-dose large volume parenteral solution – large volume parenteral solutions (e.g., containers of solution of at least 1000 mL) routinely used for compounding sterile TPN preparations or for batch compounding (e.g., sterile water for injection (SWFI); 5%, 10%, and 70% dextrose in SWFI; 0.9% sodium chloride; 0.45% sodium chloride; 5% dextrose/0.9% sodium chloride; 5% dextrose/0.45% sodium chloride)

Single-dose vial – a vial intended for a single use

Soft copy – an electronic document that is readable with the use of a special device (e.g., data processing system or computer)

Standing delegation order – written orders from a physician and designed for a patient population with specific diseases, disorders, health problems, or sets of symptoms, which provide authority for and a plan for use with patients presenting themselves prior to being examined or evaluated by a physician to assure that such acts are carried out correctly and are distinct from specific orders written for a particular patient

Standing medical order – written orders from a physician or the medical staff of an institution for patients which have been examined or evaluated by a physician and which are used as a guide in preparation for and carrying out medical or surgical procedures

Student-intern – a pharmacist-intern, registered with the board who is enrolled in the professional sequence of a college/school of pharmacy, has completed the first professional year and obtained a minimum of 30 credit hours of work towards a professional degree in pharmacy, and is participating in a board-approved internship program

Supportive personnel – individuals under the supervision of a pharmacist-in-charge, designated by the pharmacist-in-charge, and for whom the pharmacist-in-charge assumes legal responsibility, who function and perform under the instructions of the pharmacist-in-charge

Suspend – a license is of no further force and effect for a period of time as determined by the board

Substitution – the dispensing of a drug or a brand of drug other than the drug or brand of drug ordered or prescribed

Tech-check-tech – allowing a pharmacy technician to verify the accuracy of work performed by another pharmacy technician relating to the filling of floor stock and unit dose distribution systems for a patient admitted to the hospital if the patient's orders have previously been reviewed and approved by a pharmacist

Telepharmacy system – a system that monitors the dispensing of prescription drugs and provides for related drug use review and patient counseling services by an electronic method that shall include the use of the following types of technology:

- Audio and video
- Still image capture
- Store and forward

Terminal sterilization – the application of a lethal process, e.g., steam under pressure or autoclaving, to sealed final preparation containers for the purpose of achieving a predetermined sterility assurance level of usually less than 106, i.e., or a probability of less than one in one million of a non-sterile unit

Texas trade association – a cooperative and voluntarily joined statewide association of business or professional competitors in this state designed to assist its members and its industry or profession in dealing with mutual business or professional problems and in promoting their common interest

Therapeutic contact lens – a contact lens that contains one or more drugs and that delivers the drugs into the wearer's eye

Therapeutically equivalent – identical amounts will produce same therapeutic effect

Ultimate user – a person who obtains or possesses a prescription drug or device for the person's own use or for the use of a member of the person's household or for administering to an animal owned by the person or by a member of the person's household

Unidirectional flow – an airflow moving in a single direction in a robust and uniform manner and at sufficient speed to reproducibly sweep particles away from the critical processing or testing area

Unit dose packaging – the ordered amount of drug in a dosage form ready for administration to a particular patient, by the prescribed route at the prescribed time, and properly labeled with the name, strength, and expiration date of the drug

USP/NF – the current edition of the United States Pharmacopeia/National Formulary

Warehouseman – a person who stores dangerous drugs for others and who has no control over the disposition of the drugs except for the purpose of storage

Wholesaler – a person engaged in the business of distributing dangerous drugs

Written protocol – a physician's order, standing medical order, standing delegation order, or other order or protocol as defined by rule of the Texas State Board of Medical Examiners

Resources/Bibliography

NAPLEX®/MPJE® – www.nabp.net

Texas State Board of Pharmacy – http://www.tsbp.state.tx.us/

Newly adopted rules/changes for the Texas State Board of Pharmacy –
http://www.tsbp.state.tx.us/rules/Adopted_Proposed.htm

MPJE® Registration Bulletin
http://www.nabp.net/programs/assets/NAPLEX-MPJE.pdf

Drugs Therapeutic Optometrists Can Prescribe
http://www.tob.state.tx.us/TOBCode.htm#SEC358

Reference of drugs therapeutic optometrists can prescribe developed by the Texas State Board of Pharmacy
http://www.tsbp.state.tx.us/files_pdf/Optometrists.pdf

Electronic Prescriptions for Controlled Substances
http://www.deadiversion.usdoj.gov/ecomm/e_rx/faq/pharmacies.htm

Items That Can Be Changed on a Schedule II Prescription
http://www.tsbp.state.tx.us/files_pdf/changes%20to%20CII%20Rxs%2010_31_08.pdf

Texas Pharmacy Act
http://www.statutes.legis.state.tx.us/?link=OC

Texas Dangerous Drug Act
http://www.statutes.legis.state.tx.us/?link=HS

Texas Pharmacy Rules (Texas Administrative Code)
http://info.sos.state.tx.us/pls/pub/readtac$ext.ViewTAC?tac_view=3&ti=22&pt=15

Federal Food, Drug, and Cosmetic Act
http://www.access.gpo.gov/uscode/title21/chapter9_.html

Texas Food, Drug, and Cosmetic Act
http://tlo2.tlc.state.tx.us/statutes/hs.toc.htm

Federal Controlled Substance Act
http://www.deadiversion.usdoj.gov/21cfr/cfr/index.html

Poison Prevention Packaging Act
http://www.cpsc.gov/cpscpub/pubs/384.pdf

Website provided by the Texas State Board of Pharmacy with links to the Texas Pharmacy Laws and Rules
http://www.tsbp.state.tx.us/rules/Links_Rules.htm

Law Review Questions

1. Prior to September 1, 2015 pharmacists can complete their minimum 20 hour sterile compounding course through an ACPE approved course or through a structured on the job training course

   a. True
   b. False

2. If a patient is admitted to an emergency room and requires a Schedule II controlled substance upon release, what is the maximum amount that can be sent home with the patient

   a. 24 hour supply
   b. 48 hour supply
   c. 3 day supply
   d. 7 day supply

3. A Class G pharmacy may have a ratio of on-site pharmacists to pharmacy technicians and pharmacy technician trainees of

   a. 1:4
   b. 1:6
   c. 1:8
   d. Unlimited

4. Compounding a sterile preparation using less than three different sterile products not located in an ISO Class 5 or better area is considered what level of risk

   a. Low risk

b. Low risk with a 12 hour beyond use date
c. Medium risk
d. High risk

5. What form is used to notify the DEA of a theft or significant loss

    a. DEA 41
    b. DEA 106
    c. DEA 222
    d. DEA 224

6. If a pharmacy is unable to complete the partial filling of a Schedule II prescription within the required interval

    a. Prescription is now void
    b. Call prescriber to notify them and get a new prescription over the phone
    c. Call prescriber to notify them and have a new prescription written
    d. A and B
    e. A and C

7. A Class II recall means

    a. Not likely to cause adverse health effects
    b. Reasonable probability that exposure will cause serious adverse health effects or death
    c. May cause temporary or medically reversible adverse health effects
    d. None of the above

8. A Class E-S pharmacy may not renew a pharmacy license unless the pharmacy has been inspected by the board or its designee within the last two years

a. True
b. False

9. What are the requirements to become a registered pharmacy technician

   a. Have/working towards a high school diploma or GED
   b. Passed board-approved pharmacy technician certification exam
   c. Granted an exemption from taking the pharmacy technician certification exam
   d. Both A and B
   e. A, B, and C

10. Multiple dose vials may be stored for how long unless otherwise indicated by the manufacturer

   a. 4 days
   b. 10 days
   c. 28 days
   d. 30 days

11. A pharmacy that does limited prescription delivery is considered which class of pharmacy

   a. Class A
   b. Class C
   c. Class G
   d. Class H

12. How often must total particulate counts be performed in the sterile compounding areas

a. Weekly
b. Monthly
c. Every 3 months
d. Every 6 months
e. Every 12 months

13. A Class H pharmacy with multiple locations only needs to have one pharmacy license issued by the board instead of a license for each location.

   a. True
   b. False

14. How often can a retail pharmacy make a request to destroy controlled substances on their premises

   a. 6 months
   b. 12 months
   c. 24 months
   d. No request necessary

15. An opened or needle punctured single-dose containers, such as bags bottles, syringes, and vials of sterile products shall be used within what time period if opened in worse than ISO Class 5 air quality

   a. 30 minutes
   b. 60 minutes
   c. 90 minutes
   d. 120 minutes

16. Class E pharmacies that fill controlled substance prescriptions for residents in Texas must either mail or submit electronically the prescription within

a. 5 days
b. 7 days
c. 10 days
d. 14 days

17. Low risk compounded sterile preparations may be stored for how long in a solid frozen state

   a. 3 days
   b. 9 days
   c. 14 days
   d. 45 days

18. Non-pharmacist personnel may not ask questions of a patient or patient's agent which are intended to screen or limit interaction with the pharmacist

   a. True
   b. False

19. How many times may a candidate retake the MPJE

   a. Once
   b. Twice
   c. Thrice
   d. Unlimited

20. All DEA registrants are required to register every

   a. 1 year
   b. 2 years
   c. 3 years
   d. 6 months

21. High risk compounded sterile preparations may be stored for how long at room temperature

    a. 12 hours
    b. 24 hours
    c. 30 hours
    d. 48 hours

22. Which class or classes of pharmacy is required to have a perpetual inventory of Schedule II controlled substances

    a. Class A
    b. Class C
    c. Class D
    d. A and B

23. If good manufacturing principles are not followed, then drugs are considered

    a. Adultered
    b. Misbranded
    c. Both A and B

24. How many hours of vaccine-related continuing education must a pharmacist complete to maintain their vaccine administration certification

    a. 3 hours every 2 years
    b. 3 hours every year
    c. 6 hours every 2 years
    d. 6 hours every year

25. Which of the following is true regarding DEA 222 forms

I. Name and address of the supplier must be filled in
II. The number of lines completed must be filled in at the bottom
III. More than one item can be listed per line
IV. Must be completed in ink, indelible pencil, or typewritten

    a. I only
    b. I and II
    c. I, II, and IV
    d. I, II, III, and IV

26. Which of the following are required on the prescription label

I. Beyond-use date
II. Prescriber name
III. Prescriber telephone number
IV. Quantity dispensed

    a. I, III, and IV
    b. I, II, and IV
    c. II, III, and IV
    d. I, II, III, and IV

27. How often must clinic pharmacies with expanded formularies perform retrospective drug regimen reviews

    a. Monthly
    b. Bi-monthly
    c. Quarterly
    d. Annually

28. Faxed Schedule II prescriptions are allowed for

I. Narcotic for a long-term care facility patient
II. Non-narcotic for a long-term care facility patient
III. Non-narcotic for a hospice or terminally ill patient
IV. Narcotic for a hospice or terminally ill patient

a. II and III
b. I and IV
c. I, II, and IV
d. I, II, III, and IV

29. A pharmacist may dispense an electronic prescription for a Schedule II, III, IV or V controlled substance in compliance with the federal and state laws

a. True
b. False

30. Prepackaged drugs for outpatient use by a Class F pharmacy may only be dispensed for how many days

a. 24 hours
b. 48 hours
c. 72 hours
d. 96 hours

31. A licensed facility member may access an emergency medication kit during an emergency without a prescription drug order from a practitioner

a. True
b. False

32. If a supplier cannot fill the Schedule II order, how long do they have to supply the balance

    a. 14 days
    b. 30 days
    c. 60 days
    d. 90 days

33. When does a pharmacist notify a patient's primary care provider after administration of a vaccine

    a. 24 hours
    b. 5 days
    c. 7 days
    d. 10 days
    e. 14 days

34. How long may a Class H pharmacy keep prescriptions ready for a patient

    a. 7 days
    b. 10 days
    c. 15 days
    d. 30 days

35. Media fill testing is required to be done how often for high risk sterile compounding

    a. Every 6 months
    b. Every 12 months
    c. Every 24 months
    d. Not required

36. Pharmacists may now receive credit for completing Continuing Medical Education approved by the American Medical Association

    a. True
    b. False

37. What is the limit of the number of dosage units that may be prescribed at one time for multiple CII prescriptions

    a. No limit
    b. 30 dosage units
    c. 60 dosage units
    d. 90 dosage units

38. What form is used to register with the DEA

    a. DEA 41
    b. DEA 106
    c. DEA 222
    d. DEA 224

39. Air sampling in the sterile compounding areas shall be performed at least

    a. Daily
    b. Weekly
    c. Monthly
    d. Every 3 months
    e. Every 6 months
    f. Every 12 months

40. Is DEA registration number BS5383928 valid

    a. Yes

b. No

41. Which class(es) of pharmacy can outsource to a Class G pharmacy

    a. Class A
    b. Class C
    c. Class E
    d. Class G
    e. A, B and C
    f. A and C
    g. A and D

42. Pharmacy technicians are allowed to transfer controlled substance prescriptions orally between pharmacies

    a. True
    b. False

43. Low risk compounded sterile preparations may be stored for how long at cold/refrigerated temperature

    a. 2 days
    b. 9 days
    c. 14 days
    d. 45 days

44. The student-intern card issued by the board expires when the student-intern

    I. Ceases enrollment in school
    II. Fails the NAPLEX® and/or MPJE® examinations
    III. Fails to take the NAPLEX® and/or MPJE® within 6 calendar months after graduation

IV.   Fail to take the NAPLEX® and/or MPJE® within
       3 calendar months after graduation

       a. I and III
       b. I and IV
       c. I, II, III
       d. I, II, and IV

45. Media fill testing is required to be done how often for
     low and medium risk sterile compounding

       a. Every 6 months
       b. Every 12 months
       c. Every 24 months
       d. Not required

46. Controlled substances are not allowed to be in an
     emergency medication kit

       a. True
       b. False

47. If a prescription has been misfiled (substituted in whole
     or in part), then it is considered

       a. Adultered
       b. Misbranded
       c. Both A and B

48. A patient that has been treated in the emergency room
     requires an emergency quantity of a Schedule III
     controlled substance upon discharge, what is the
     maximum-day supply that can be dispensed

       a. 3 days

b. 7 days
c. 10 days
d. 14 days
e. Amount determined appropriate by the prescriber until the patient can reach a pharmacy

49. Which of the following cannot be dispensed from a Class D pharmacy

a. Anti-infective drugs
b. Musculoskeletal drugs
c. Erectile dysfunction drugs
d. Obstetrical and gynecological drugs

50. Exposing the sterile ingredients and components used to prepare and package compounded sterile preparations to room air quality worse than ISO Class 5 is considered what level of risk

a. Low risk
b. Low risk with a 12 hour beyond use date
c. Medium risk
d. High risk

51. Who is allowed to sign or execute a DEA 222 form

a. Individual who signed the DEA registration
b. Individual or individuals who signed a Power of Attorney from the individual who signed the DEA registration
c. Owner and also the pharmacist in charge
d. A and B

52. What is the maximum-day supply a physician can issue for multiple CII prescriptions

    a. 30 days
    b. 60 days
    c. 90 days
    d. No maximum

53. A Class D pharmacy may dispense prescriptions to patients other than those at the clinic where the pharmacy is located

    a. True
    b. False

54. Can an order for Schedule II controlled substances be shipped to a different location than what is listed on the DEA 222 form

    a. No
    b. Yes

55. How many temporary locations can a clinic pharmacy operate at one time

    a. Two
    b. Three
    c. Four
    d. Six

56. A patient that has been treated in the emergency room requires an emergency quantity of a Schedule II controlled substance upon discharge. What is the maximum-day supply that can be dispensed

a. 3 days
b. 5 days
c. 7 days
d. 10 days

57. The pharmacist-in-charge for a Class H pharmacy must be employed at least full-time

   a. True
   b. False

58. An authorized agent of the prescriber may

   I. Prepare a controlled substance prescription for the signature of the prescriber
   II. Orally communicate a prescriber's Schedule III–V prescription to a pharmacist
   III. Transmit by fax a prescriber's written Schedule II prescription to a pharmacist
   IV. Orally communicate a prescriber's emergency Schedule II prescription to a pharmacist

   a. I only
   b. I and II
   c. I, II, and III
   d. I, II, III, and IV

59. The pseudoephedrine and ephedrine laws in Texas do not apply to the liquid, liquid capsule, or liquid gel capsule form

   a. True
   b. False

60. If a pharmacist fills a prescription without authorization from the prescriber, it is considered

   a. Adultered
   b. Misbranded
   c. Both A and B

61. At each step of the compounding process, the pharmacist shall ensure that components used in compounding are accurately weighed, measured, or subdivided as appropriate to conform to the formula being prepared

   a. True
   b. False

62. A patient has a prescription for clonazepam 1 mg tablet by mouth twice daily #60 with 3 refills. The patient only wants to receive 20 tablets at a time. What is the total quantity that can be filled with this prescription if the patient only gets 20 tablets at a time within a 6-month time period

   a. 60 tablets
   b. 120 tablets
   c. 180 tablets
   d. 240 tablets

63. Which copy of the DEA 222 form does the purchaser keep for their records

   a. Copy 1
   b. Copy 2
   c. Copy 3

64. Medium risk compounded sterile preparations may be stored for how long in a solid frozen state

    a. 3 days
    b. 9 days
    c. 14 days
    d. 45 days

65. Which copy of the DEA 222 form does the supplier send to the DEA

    a. Copy 1
    b. Copy 2
    c. Copy 3

66. Which classes of pharmacy are allowed to provide emergency medication kits

    a. Class A
    b. Class B
    c. Class C
    d. Class D
    e. Class E
    f. Class A and C
    g. Class A and E
    h. Class A, C and E
    i. Class A, D and E

67. The pharmacist-in-charge for a Class H pharmacy may only be the pharmacist-in-charge for one Class H pharmacy

    a. True
    b. False

68.   A pharmacy located in a free standing emergency center is considered which class of pharmacy

      a. Class D
      b. Class E
      c. Class F
      d. Class G
      e. Class H

69.   How often does a pharmacy prescription balance need to be inspected

      a. Every year
      b. Every two years
      c. Every three years
      d. Doesn't need to be inspected

70.   If a pharmacy is allowed to partial fill a Schedule II prescription, within what time frame are they required to supply the remainder

      a. 24 hours
      b. 48 hours
      c. 72 hours
      d. 96 hours

71.   How many hours of instruction and experience are required for pharmacy technicians to compound sterile preparations

      a. 10 hours
      b. 20 hours
      c. 40 hours
      d. 50 hours

72. The only way a prescriber can specify the dispensing of a brand drug product is to handwrite on the prescription "brand necessary" or "brand medically necessary"

    a. True
    b. False

73. A Class A pharmacy may use an auto-refill program for which of the following

    I.   Dangerous drugs
    II.   Schedule II
    III.   Schedule III
    IV.   Schedule IV
    V.   Schedule V

    a. I only
    b. I, III, IV, V
    c. I, II, III, IV, V
    d. I, IV, and V

74. How many members make up the Texas State Board of Pharmacy

    a. 7
    b. 8
    c. 9
    d. 10
    e. 11

75. Effective September 1, 2015, how many hours of continuing education related to compounding sterile preparations are required for their registration renewal

if the pharmacy technician is engaged in compounding high risk sterile preparations

    a. One
    b. Two
    c. Four
    d. Six

76. When compounding is done by a pharmacy technician, the pharmacist has to supervise the technician and conduct in-process and final checks.

    a. True
    b. False

77. A pharmacist-in-charge can only be the pharmacist-in-charge for one Class D pharmacy

    a. True
    b. False

78. The pharmacist-in-charge of a Class G pharmacy may be the pharmacist-in-charge for more than one Glass G pharmacy

    a. True
    b. False

79. If the strength of the prescription drug does not meet what it says on the label, then it is considered

    a. Adultered
    b. Misbranded
    c. A and B

80. When do you have to notify the DPS about any change in business name or address

    a. Within 7 days
    b. Within 10 days
    c. Within 14 days
    d. Within 30 days

81. In the buffer area, ante-area, and segregated compounding area, walls, ceilings, and shelving shall be cleaned and disinfected

    a. Daily
    b. Weekly
    c. Monthly
    d. Bi-annually

82. Who is responsible for all the administrative and operational functions of a Class D pharmacy

    a. Pharmacist-in-charge
    b. Consultant pharmacist
    c. Staff pharmacist
    d. Owner

83. When partial filling a Schedule II for a long-term care facility resident, for how long is the prescription good, from the day it was written

    a. 10 days
    b. 21 days
    c. 30 days
    d. 60 days

84. Which inventory(s) do NOT have to be notarized by the pharmacist-in-charge within 72 hours or three working days of completing the inventory

    a. Initial
    b. Annual
    c. Change of ownership
    d. Closing
    e. All of the above

85. A pharmacist can only administer a vaccine upon referral from a physician who has an established physician-patient relationship to a patient that is under 14 years old

    a. True
    b. False

86. Who is responsible for the practice of pharmacy at a Class G pharmacy

    a. Owner
    b. Pharmacist-in-charge
    c. Staff pharmacist
    d. Lead pharmacy technician

87. A medication that is compounded only using single volume transfers within an ISO Class 5 environment has a beyond-use date at a cold temperature (refrigerated) of

    a. 14 days
    b. 9 days
    c. 3 days
    d. 1 day

88. A compounded total parentral nutrition fluid has a beyond-use date at room temperature of no more than

    a. 12 hours
    b. 24 hours
    c. 30 hours
    d. 48 hours

89. How often should environmental testing be conducted at a minimum for compounding sterile preparations

    a. Weekly
    b. Monthly
    c. Every 3 months
    d. Every 6 months
    e. Every 12 months

90. A FEMCC pharmacy shall maintain a perpetual inventory of any controlled substance listed in Schedule II

    a. True
    b. False

91. How often must the pharmacist-in-charge, consultant pharmacist, or staff pharmacist shall personally visit the Class H pharmacy

    a. At least weekly
    b. At least bi-weekly
    c. At least monthly
    d. At least bi-monthly

92. Electronic prescriptions are allowed for practitioners licensed in Canada or Mexico

    a. True
    b. False

93. The pharmacist-in-charge of a Class D pharmacy must be employed on a full-time basis

    a. True
    b. False

94. What is the minimum age of a patient may a pharmacist to administer an influenza vaccine without a physician-patient relationship

    a. 3 years old
    b. 5 years old
    c. 7 years old
    d. 14 years old

95. Medium risk compounded sterile preparations may be stored for how long at room temperature

    a. 12 hours
    b. 24 hours
    c. 30 hours
    d. 48 hours

96. An official prescription form for a Schedule II controlled substance is not required for a(n)

    I.   Inmate at a correctional facility
    II.   Animal admitted to an animal hospital
    III. Patient admitted to a hospital

IV.   Patient receiving a medication from an emergency kit at a long term care facility

     a. I and II
     b. I, II, and III
     c. II, III, and IV
     d. I, II, III, and IV

97.   How many hours of continuing education are required to renew a pharmacist's license

     a. 15 hours
     b. 20 hours
     c. 30 hours
     d. 40 hours

98.   Class E pharmacies cannot dispense prescriptions for controlled substances to patients in this state even if written by a prescriber registered with the Texas Department of Safety

     a. True
     b. False

99.   Both the patient's and prescriber's name and address must be present on a controlled substance prescription

     a. True
     b. False

100. When transferring Schedule II controlled substances between pharmacies, which form is used

     a. DEA 41
     b. DEA 106

c. DEA 222
d. No form required

101. When does a retail pharmacy have to make a request to destroy controlled substances on their premises

a. 7 days prior
b. 10 days prior
c. 14 days prior
d. No request necessary

102. If a pharmacist does not have malpractice insurance and a claim or complaint is filed against them, when do they have to notify the board

a. Within 10 days
b. Within 14 days
c. Within 30 days
d. Within 60 days

103. Physicians are allowed to write controlled substance prescriptions "for office use"

a. True
b. False

104. If you fail the NAPLEX®, how many times can you retake the test

a. One time
b. Two times
c. Three times
d. Unlimited

105. Class D pharmacies are allowed to dispense Schedule IV and V controlled substances but not Schedule I, II, or III

    a. True
    b. False

106. Compounding a sterile preparation to be infused over several days at room temperature is considered what level of risk

    a. Low risk
    b. Low risk with a 12 hour beyond use date
    c. Medium risk
    d. High risk

107. Where must the approval certificate for providing emergency medication kits be displayed

    a. Provider pharmacy
    b. Remote site
    c. Does not need to be displayed

108. A non-resident pharmacy is considered which class of pharmacy

    a. Class D
    b. Class E
    c. Class F
    d. Class G
    e. Class H

109. When does a pharmacy have to notify the Texas Department of Public Safety about a discrepancy or theft

a. As soon as possible
b. Within 24 hours
c. Within 48 hours
d. Within 96 hours

110. Which of the following are required on a Schedule II prescription

I.   Patient's address
II.   Prescriber's address
III. Prescriber's phone number

    a. I, II, and III
    b. I and II
    c. II and III
    d. I and III
    e. II only

111. If a patient does not pick up a prescription at a Class H pharmacy, the pharmacy can return the medications to stock to be reused

    a. True
    b. False

112. When a registrant changes their business name or address, when does the Texas Department of Public Safety have to be notified

    a. Within 5 days
    b. Within 7 days
    c. Within 10 days
    d. Within 14 days

113. How many hours of instruction and experience are required for pharmacists to compound sterile preparations

    a. 10 hours
    b. 20 hours
    c. 40 hours
    d. 50 hours

114. Immediate use compounded sterile preparations may only be made with how many products including an infusion or diluent solution

    a. One
    b. Two
    c. Three
    d. Four

115. The board of pharmacy may not inspect which of the following without consent

    a. Financial data
    b. Shipment data
    c. Pricing data
    d. A and B
    e. A and C
    f. A, B, and C

116. A practitioner may only prescribe methadone for the maintenance or detoxification of opioid addicted individuals if they are registered with the DEA as a Narcotic Treatment Program

    a. True
    b. False

117. How often must the pharmacist-in-charge, staff pharmacist, or consultant pharmacist personally visit the clinic pharmacy

    a. Weekly
    b. Every two weeks
    c. Monthly
    d. Every two months

118. If the packaging on a prescription violates the Poison Prevention Packaging Act, then it is considered

    a. Adultered
    b. Misbranded
    c. Both A and B

119. A Class D pharmacy that operates a temporary location may leave prescriptions for patients to pick up later as long as they are dangerous drugs only and not controlled substances

    a. True
    b. False

120. Which class or classes of pharmacy are required to have a perpetual inventory of Schedule I and IIs

    a. Class A
    b. Class B
    c. Class C
    d. Both A and C

121. How many hours of training must a pharmacist complete before becoming certified to administer vaccines

    a. 10 hours
    b. 20 hours
    c. 30 hours
    d. 40 hours

122. How many hours of training must a pharmacist who works in a Class B pharmacy complete

    a. 500 hours
    b. 700 hours
    c. 1,000 hours
    d. 1,500 hours

123. How long is a temporary pharmacist license for an active duty military spouse valid for unless extended by the board

    a. Two months
    b. Three months
    c. Four months
    d. Six months

124. What form is used when transferring Schedule IIIs between pharmacies

    a. Invoice only
    b. DEA 106
    c. DEA 41
    d. DEA 222

125. In order to process electronic controlled substance prescriptions, pharmacies must use specific software approved by the DEA, which must be certified by a third party audit

    a. True
    b. False

126. Both the pharmacist and the physician are required to have their signatures on Schedule II prescriptions

    a. True
    b. False

127. If a pharmacist has malpractice insurance and a claim or complaint is filed against the pharmacist, who is responsible for notifying the board

    a. Pharmacist
    b. Insurance company

128. A temporary pharmacist license may be granted for a pharmacist seeking a reciprocity license with an active duty military spouse prior to taking the Texas MPJE

    a. True
    b. False

129. What is the maximum number of internship hours that can be counted per week

    a. 40 hours
    b. 50 hours
    c. 60 hours
    d. 30 hours

130. If a hospital pharmacy does not have a pharmacist on-site, who is allowed to remove medications from the pharmacy

    a. Licensed nurse
    b. Practitioner
    c. Nurse aide
    d. A and B

131. When a physician orally communicates a Schedule II controlled substance prescription to a pharmacist, what is the maximum-day supply that is allowed to be dispensed

    a. 1 day
    b. 2 days
    c. 3 days
    d. Quantity necessary to treat the patient during the emergency period

132. The initials of the pharmacist providing the counseling for each prescription needs to be documented

    a. True
    b. False

133. Compounding a sterile preparation using less than three different sterile products in an ISO Class 5 or better area is considered what level of risk

    a. Low risk
    b. Low risk with a 12 hour beyond use date
    c. Medium risk
    d. High risk

134. When does a pharmacist notify the physician in the written protocol after administration of a vaccine

    a. 24 hours
    b. 48 hours
    c. 7 days
    d. 10 day

135. What information must be recorded when delivering controlled substances either by an authorized delivery person or by mail and how long must the record be maintained

    I.   Name of the authorized delivery person
    II.   Mailing address
    III.   2 years
    IV.   3 years

    a. I, II, and III
    b. I, II, and IV
    c. I and III
    d. I and IV

136. What are the prescription label requirements for a cat

    a. Cat's name
    b. Owner's name
    c. Species
    d. A and B
    e. B and C
    f. A, B, and C

137. Withdrawals from a closed Class F pharmacy with a full-time pharmacist must be verified within

a. 24 hours
b. 48 hours
c. 72 hours
d. 96 hours

138. A Class E pharmacy may use an auto-refill program for which of the following

I.   Dangerous drugs
II.   Schedule II
III. Schedule III
IV.   Schedule IV
V.   Schedule V

a. I only
b. I, III, IV, V
c. I, II, III, IV, V
d. I, IV, and V

139. There can be multiple prescriptions written for Schedule IIs as long as they are on the same official prescription form

a. True
b. False

140. Which of the following are required on the prescription label

I.   Pharmacy address
II.   Pharmacy telephone number
III. Date prescription dispensed
IV.   Date prescription written

a. II, III, and IV
b. II and IV
c. I, II, and III
d. I, II, III, and IV

141. Pharmacists may not transfer their sterile compounding training to another pharmacy unless the pharmacies are under common ownership and control and use a common training program

a. True
b. False

142. When do intern hours expire after completion of the internship

a. 6 months
b. 1 year
c. 18 months
d. 2 years

143. Who is responsible for the administrative and operational concerns of a Class G pharmacy

a. Owner
b. Pharmacist-in-charge
c. Staff pharmacist
d. Lead pharmacy technician

144. A Class C pharmacy with fewer than 100 beds needs to have which of the following

a. Part-time pharmacist
b. Consulting pharmacist

c. Continuous on-site pharmacist
d. A or B

145. Which filling system for prescriptions and other records is required in Texas

    a. Schedule I, Schedule II, Schedule III–V, and dangerous drugs
    b. Schedule I and II, Schedule III–V and dangerous drugs
    c. Schedule I–V, and dangerous drugs

146. How long must records be kept at a Class H pharmacy

    a. One year
    b. Two years
    c. Three years
    d. Four years

147. In a Class A pharmacy, any consultation with the prescriber must be recorded onto the hard-copy or in the data processing system with the pharmacist's initials

    a. True
    b. False

148. A Schedule II prescription must be filled no later than how many days after the date of issuance

    a. 7 days
    b. 10 days
    c. 14 days
    d. 21 days

149. How often does a controlled substance inventory need to occur

    a. Every 6 months
    b. Every year
    c. Every 2 years
    d. Not required

150. A provider pharmacy for remote pharmacy services for emergency kits must be located within how many miles from the facility the emergency kit is kept

    a. 10 miles
    b. 20 miles
    c. 50 miles
    d. Provider pharmacy may be any distance

151. Effective September 1, 2015, how many hours of continuing education related to compounding sterile preparations are required for their registration renewal if the pharmacy technician is engaged in compounding low and medium risk sterile preparations

    a. One
    b. Two
    c. Four
    d. Six

152. What form is used when transferring Schedule III, IV, and Vs between pharmacies

    a. Invoice only
    b. DEA 106
    c. DEA 41
    d. DEA 222

153. Pharmacists may now receive credit for completing Continuing Medical Education approved by the American Medical Association

    a. True
    b. False

154. A physician who is not registered to conduct a narcotic treatment program may administer narcotic drugs to relieve acute withdrawal symptoms. However, the emergency treatment may only be carried out for one day

    a. True
    b. False

155. How is the president of the board decided

    a. Elected by the board
    b. Elected by the voters
    c. Appointed by the senate
    d. Appointed by the governor

156. If a pharmacist's license has been revoked, after how long can they reapply to the board

    a. 6 months
    b. 12 months
    c. 24 months
    d. Never

157. When a pharmacy closes, what form do they use to transfer Schedule IIs to another pharmacy?

a. DEA 41
b. DEA 106
c. DEA 222
d. No form required

158. How long must you keep continuing education records

    a. 1 year
    b. 2 years
    c. 3 years
    d. 4 years

159. Dissolving non-sterile bulk drug powders to make solutions, which will be terminally sterilized is considered what level of risk

    a. Low risk
    b. Low risk with a 12 hour beyond use date
    c. Medium risk
    d. High risk

160. Cleaning and disinfecting the sterile compounding area shall occur at a minimum of

    a. Prior to and after each work shift
    b. Every 12 hours
    c. After spills
    d. All of the above

161. How long are the terms for board members

    a. 2 years
    b. 4 years
    c. 5 years
    d. 6 years

162. Which of the following can be done by a pharmacist only and not a pharmacy technician

    a. Entering prescription order information into the data processing system
    b. Initiating and receiving refill authorization requests
    c. Communicating to the patient information concerning any prescription drugs dispensed to the patient by the pharmacy

163. If a pharmacist signs a prescription for a dangerous drug under the delegated authority of a prescriber then the pharmacist's name must appear on the label of the prescription

    a. True
    b. False

164. How many gloved fingertip/thumb samplings are required before being allowed to compound sterile preparations for patient use

    a. One
    b. Two
    c. Three
    d. Four

165. When does the DEA have to be notified prior to a transfer of business

    a. 1 day
    b. 7 days
    c. 10 days

d. 14 days

166. Board must be notified of a change in schedule of operation of a clinic pharmacy (Class D)

    a. True
    b. False

167. What is the minimum age a person can be in order to purchase a pseudoephedrine product

    a. 16 years old
    b. 18 years old
    c. 21 years old
    d. No age requirement

168. The prescriber's DPS number and DEA number are required on a Schedule II prescription

    a. True
    b. False

169. Which of the following is required to be recorded from a purchaser of pseudoephedrine products

    a. Name
    b. Address
    c. Date of birth
    d. Identification number
    e. All of the above

170. If a pharmacist determines that it is in the best interest of the patient to provide an emergency refill of a dangerous drug without prescriber authorization, what is the maximum supply that can be dispensed

a. 24 hours
b. 48 hours
c. 36 hours
d. 72 hours
e. No limit

171. How many hours of continuing education are required for pharmacy technicians to renew their registration

a. 10 hours
b. 20 hours
c. 30 hours
d. None

172. When a pharmacy will be transferring their business and their Schedule II controlled substances, when does the DEA have to be notified

a. 7 days prior
b. 14 days prior
c. 10 days after
d. 14 days after
e. 7 days after

173. Which of the following are true regarding pharmacist preceptor requirements

I. Minimum of 1 year as a licensed pharmacist
II. Active pharmacist license
III. Complete 3 hours of preceptor training initially
IV. Complete 3 hours of preceptor training during each license renewal period

a. I and III

b. II, III, and IV

c. I, II, and III

d. I, II, III, and IV

174. What is the ratio of pharmacists to pharmacy technicians in a Class A pharmacy that dispenses more than 20 different prescription drugs

a. 1:1

b. 1:2

c. 1:3

d. 1:4

e. Unlimited

175. Which of the following are allowed to be prescribed by therapeutic optometrists

a. 4-day supply of a Schedule III

b. 10-day supply of antibiotics

c. 10-day supply of non-steroidal anti-inflammatories

d. 7-day supply of antihistamines

176. Over-the-counter drug advertising is regulated by

a. FDA

b. Federal Trade Commission

c. Department of Public Safety

d. DEA

177. The name of the advanced practice nurse or physician assistant and the name of the supervising physician are required to be on the prescription label

a. True

b. False

178. Prior to September 1, 2015 all pharmacists engaged in compounding sterile preparations shall obtain continuing education appropriate for the type of compounding done by the pharmacist

   a. True
   b. False

179. If a pharmacy doesn't have the full quantity of a Schedule II to fill a prescription, are they allowed to partial fill it

   a. Yes
   b. No

180. What is the minimum time you have to wait to retake the NAPLEX® or MPJE® if you failed

   a. 30 days
   b. 60 day
   c. 90 days

181. How many hours of continuing education must a pharmacist complete in their initial license period

   a. 10 hours
   b. 15 hours
   c. 30 hours
   d. None

182. Which of the following MAY be changed on a Schedule II prescription

I.   Name of the drug
II.   Strength of the drug
III.   Date of the prescription
IV.   Name of the prescriber

    a. I and II
    b. II only
    c. II and III
    d. I, II, III, and IV

183. Drugs cannot be removed when a Class F pharmacy with a full-time pharmacist is closed

    a. True
    b. False

184. Effective September 1, 2015, how many hours of continuing education related to compounding sterile preparations are required for their license renewal if the pharmacist is engaged in compounding low and medium risk sterile preparations

    a. One
    b. Two
    c. Four
    d. Six

185. What class or schedule of drug is carisoprodol listed in

    a. Dangerous drug
    b. Schedule V
    c. Schedule IV
    d. Schedule III

186. The pharmacist-in-charge of a Class G pharmacy has to be employed full time at that pharmacy

    a. True
    b. False

187. An electronic transfer between pharmacies may be initiated by a pharmacist intern, pharmacy technician, or pharmacy technician trainee acting under the direct supervision of a pharmacist

    a. True
    b. False

188. Which of the following requires the continuous presence of a pharmacist during business hours

    a. Class A
    b. Class B
    c. Class C with more than 100 beds
    d. A and C
    e. All of the above

189. Pharmacy technician trainees may begin work prior to registering with the Texas State Board of Pharmacy

    a. True
    b. False

190. If a pharmacist determines that providing an emergency refill of a Schedule III controlled substance is appropriate, what is the maximum supply that can be dispensed

    a. 24 hours

b. 48 hours
c. 72 hours
d. 96 hours

191. Which of the following are true regarding partial filling a Schedule II prescription for a terminally ill or long-term care facility resident

    I.   Must have "terminally ill" or "long-term care facility resident" on the face of the prescription

    II.   Can only partially fill a prescription 5 times

    III.   Pharmacist must write on the back of the prescription: date of the dispensing, quantity dispensed, quantity remaining, and identification of the pharmacist

    IV.   Prescription is valid for 60 days from date of issue

    a. I and IV
    b. I, III, and IV
    c. II, III, and IV
    d. I, II, III, and IV

192. The 1906 Pure Food and Drug Act requires which standard for drugs

    a. Purity
    b. Efficacy
    c. Safety

193. When do you have to notify the board about loss of data

    a. Immediately
    b. 1 day
    c. 10 days

d. 14 days

194. After telephoning in an emergency Schedule II prescription to a pharmacy, the prescriber has how many days to send in the official written prescription

   a. 3 days
   b. 7 days
   c. 10 days
   d. 14 days

195. Filling of reservoirs of injection and infusion devices with multiple sterile drug products, and evacuating air from those reservoirs before the filled device is dispensed is considered what level of risk

   a. Low risk
   b. Low risk with a 12 hour beyond use date
   c. Medium risk
   d. High risk

196. If a patient is admitted to the hospital for a surgical procedure, prescribers are allowed to maintain or detoxify the patient using narcotic drugs with having to be registered with the Narcotic Treatment Program

   a. True
   b. False

197. How long do media-fill tests need to be incubated

   a. 5 days
   b. 7 days
   c. 10 days
   d. 14 days

198. How much of the total number of controlled substances dispensed in a year may a pharmacy transfer without having to register as a wholesaler

    a. 2%
    b. 5%
    c. 10%
    d. 20%

199. Withdrawals from a closed Class F pharmacy with only a consultant pharmacist must be verified within

    a. 72 hours
    b. 96 hours
    c. 7 days
    d. 10 days

200. A provider pharmacy must apply to the board to provide remote pharmacy services using an emergency medication kit

    a. True
    b. False

201. Measuring and mixing sterile ingredients in non-sterile devices before sterilization is performed is considered what level of risk

    a. Low risk
    b. Low risk with a 12 hour beyond use date
    c. Medium risk
    d. High risk

202. How are the members of the Board determined

a. Appointed by the governor
b. Appointed by the senate
c. Elected by the citizens of Texas
d. Appointed by the House of Representatives

203. A pharmacist may not add flavoring to an over-the-counter product at the request of a patient or patient's agent unless the pharmacist obtains a prescription for the over-the-counter product from the patient's practitioner

a. True
b. False

204. Prescribers are not allowed to prescribe methadone for pain unless they are registered with the DEA as a Narcotic Treatment Program

a. True
b. False

205. Compounding records need to be kept at the pharmacy for a minimum of

a. One year
b. Two years
c. Three years
d. Don't need to be kept

206. Within how many days must a student-intern report a change of employment to the board

a. 14 days
b. 10 days

c. 7 days

d. Not necessary to inform the board

207. When is the DEA required to be notified after a theft or significant loss

    a. One business day
    b. Immediately
    c. 7 days
    d. 10 days

208. Pharmacy personnel who fail written tests or whose media-fill test vials result in gross microbial colonization may continue to compound sterile preparations until they pass the written test or media-fill test

    a. True
    b. False

209. A Schedule II controlled substance prescription must be filled not later than how many days after the date of issuance

    a. 7 days
    b. 10 days
    c. 14 days
    d. 21 days

210. The pharmacist-in-charge for the Class E pharmacy must be licensed in

    a. Texas
    b. The state the Class E pharmacy is physically located

c. Any state
d. Both A and B

211. How many hours of coursework are required to become a student-intern

    a. None
    b. 15 hours
    c. 20 hours
    d. 30 hours

212. How many hours of drug therapy–related continuing education must a pharmacist that performs drug therapy management under a physician protocol complete each year

    a. 3 hours every year
    b. 3 hours every 2 years
    c. 6 hours every year
    d. 6 hours every 2 years

213. A student intern may transfer a dangerous drug prescription to another student intern in a Class A pharmacy

    a. True
    b. False

214. Registration with the Texas Department of Public Safety occurs every

    a. 6 months
    b. 12 months
    c. 24 months
    d. 36 months

215. In a rural hospital when a pharmacist is not on duty and a nurse withdraws a medication from the pharmacy, when must the pharmacist verify the withdrawal

    a. Within 24 hours
    b. Within 2 days
    c. Within 5 days
    d. Within 7 days

216. Human growth hormone and anabolic steroids are listed as

    a. Dangerous drugs
    b. Schedule V
    c. Schedule IV
    d. Schedule III

217. Medium risk compounded sterile preparations may be stored for how long at cold/refrigerated temperature

    a. 2 days
    b. 9 days
    c. 14 days
    d. 45 days

218. Prescription drug advertising is regulated by the

    a. FDA
    b. Federal Trade Commission
    c. Department of Public Safety
    d. DEA

219. Which class(es) of pharmacy can outsource to a Class H pharmacy

a. Class A
b. Class C
c. Class E
d. Class G
e. A and C
f. A and D

220. The "tech-check-tech" program, which allows pharmacy technicians to perform checking duties without a pharmacist's verification, is allowed in which class or classes of pharmacy

a. Class A
b. Class C
c. Class B
d. Both Class A and Class B pharmacies

221. When a retail pharmacy requests permission to destroy controlled substances, what form must they send to the DEA

a. DEA 41
b. DEA 106
c. DEA 222
d. No form required

222. The 1938 Federal Food, Drug and Cosmetic Act requires which standard for drugs

a. Purity
b. Efficacy
c. Safety

223. When performing an inventory of controlled substances, which of the following are true

I.   Actual count of Schedule II
II.   Estimated count of Schedule III, IV, V if container holds <1,000 units
III.   Actual count of Schedule III, IV, V if container holds >1,000 units
IV.   Actual count of Schedule III, IV, V if container holds <1,000 units

    a. I only
    b. I and II
    c. I, III, and IV
    d. I, II, and III

223. The 1962 Kefauver-Harris Amendment required which standard for drugs

    a. Purity
    b. Efficacy
    c. Safety

224. What is the minimum age a woman must be to purchase Plan B without a prescription

    a. 14
    b. 15
    c. 16
    d. 17
    e. 18

225. How often do you have to register with the Texas Department of Public Safety (DPS)

a. Every 6 months
b. Every year
c. Every two years
d. Every three years

226. A provider pharmacy may provide remote emergency medication kits at more than one remote site

a. True
b. False

227. Which Act or Amendment created over-the-counter and prescription drug classifications

a. Federal Food, Drug and Cosmetic Act
b. Kefauver-Harris Amendment
c. Durham-Humphrey Amendments
d. Pure Food and Drug Act

228. Which of the following are required on the prescription label

I. Pharmacy address
II. Pharmacy telephone number
III. Date prescription dispensed
IV. Date prescription written

a. II, III, and IV
b. II and IV
c. I, II, and III
d. I, II, III, and IV

229. What is the ratio of pharmacists to pharmacy technicians in a Class B pharmacy

a. 1:1
b. 1:2
c. 1:3
d. 1:4
e. Unlimited

230. Effective September 1, 2015 pharmacists can complete their minimum 20 hour sterile compounding course through an ACPE approved course or through a structured on the job training course

a. True
b. False

231. What is the ratio of pharmacists to pharmacy technicians in a Class A pharmacy that dispenses no more than 20 different medications

a. 1:1
b. 1:2
c. 1:3
d. 1:5
e. Unlimited

232. A Class H pharmacy may not deliver prescription drug orders for controlled substances

a. True
b. False

233. Single-dose containers, including single-dose large volume parenteral solutions and single-dose vials, exposed to ISO Class 5 or cleaner air may be used up to how long after initial needle puncture

a. 1 hour
b. 2 hours
c. 4 hours
d. 6 hours
e. 8 hours

234. How long can someone be a pharmacy technician trainee

a. 90 days
b. 1 year
c. 2 years
d. Unlimited as long as registration is renewed

235. The pressure differential or airflow between the buffer area and the ante-area and between the ante-area and the general environment outside the compounding area shall be documented on the log at least

a. Daily
b. Weekly
c. Monthly
d. Every 3 months
e. Every 6 months
f. Every 12 months

236. Pharmacies must do an inventory and include which medications

a. Controlled substances
b. All dosage forms containing nalbuphine
c. Tramadol
d. All of the above

237. High risk compounded sterile preparations may be stored for how long in a solid frozen state

    a. 3 days
    b. 9 days
    c. 14 days
    d. 45 days

238. Class D pharmacies must have a formulary which lists all drugs and devices that are administered, dispensed, or provided by the Class D pharmacy

    a. True
    b. False

239. What form is submitted to the DEA when destroying controlled substances

    a. DEA 41
    b. DEA 106
    c. DEA 222
    d. DEA 224

240. A Class F pharmacy must have a pharmacist-in-charge employed on a full-time basis

    a. True
    b. False

241. Immediate use sterile compounds must be administered within what time frame from preparation

    a. 30 minutes
    b. 60 minutes
    c. 90 minutes

d. 120 minutes

242. When transferring Schedule II controlled substances to a reverse distributor for destruction, which form is used

    a. DEA 41
    b. DEA 106
    c. DEA 222
    d. No form required

243. A prescriber can specify the dispensing of a brand drug product if they sign on the line that says "brand necessary"

    a. True
    b. False

244. A pharmacist may add flavoring to a prescription at the request of a patient, the patient's agent, or the prescriber

    a. True
    b. False

245. How many times can a dangerous drug prescription be transferred if written by an out-of-state provider

    a. Once
    b. Twice
    c. Thrice
    d. Unlimited

246. Which act bans the sale, trade or purchase of prescription drug samples

a. Drug Price Competition and Patent Restoration Act
b. FDA Modernization Act
c. Orphan Drug Act
d. Prescription Drug Marketing Act

247. How many hours of CE related to Texas pharmacy laws and rules are required for pharmacist license renewal

   a. 0.5 hours
   b. 1 hour
   c. 2 hours
   d. 3 hours
   e. Not required

248. How many Class D pharmacies can a consultant pharmacist be a consultant for

   a. One
   b. Two
   c. Three
   d. Unlimited

249. Which component of sterile compounding garb can be reused if kept in the anteroom during the work shift

   a. Hair mask
   b. Face mask
   c. Shoe covers
   d. Gown
   e. Gloves
   f. All of the above

250. Low risk compounded sterile preparations may be stored for how long at room temperature

a. 12 hours
b. 24 hours
c. 30 hours
d. 48 hours

251. Can a man purchase Plan B without a prescription

a. No
b. Yes, if he is 17 years of age or older
c. Yes, if he is 18 years of age or older

252. Compounding parentral nutrition either by hand or through an automated compounder is considered what level of risk

a. Low risk
b. Low risk with a 12 hour beyond use date
c. Medium risk
d. High risk

253. High risk compounded sterile preparations may be stored for how long at cold/refrigerated temperature

a. 3 days
b. 9 days
c. 14 days
d. 45 days

254. If the labeling is false or misleading, then it is considered

a. Adultered
b. Misbranded
c. Both A and B

255. Faxed prescriptions for Schedule III-V are not allowed

    a. True
    b. False

256. Compounding a sterile preparation using more than three different sterile products is considered what level of risk

    a. Low risk
    b. Low risk with a 12 hour beyond use date
    c. Medium risk
    d. High risk

257. How many intern hours are required to become a pharmacist in Texas

    a. 500
    b. 1,000
    c. 1,250
    d. 1,500

258. Effective September 1, 2015, how many hours of continuing education related to compounding sterile preparations are required for their license renewal if the pharmacist is engaged in compounding high risk sterile preparations

    a. One
    b. Two
    c. Four
    d. Six

259. When transferring Schedule III, IV, and V controlled substances between pharmacies, which form is used

    a. DEA 41
    b. DEA 106
    c. DEA 222
    d. No form required

260. Single volume transfers of sterile dosage forms from ampules, bottles, bags, and vials; using sterile syringes with sterile needles, other administration devices, and other sterile containers is considered what level of risk

    a. Low risk
    b. Low risk with a 12 hour beyond use date
    c. Medium risk
    d. High risk

261. What is the minimum age of a patient for a pharmacist to administer a vaccine other than the influenza vaccine without a physician-patient relationship

    a. 7 years old
    b. 10 years old
    c. 14 years old
    d. 18 years old

262. How many members of the board are pharmacists

    a. 4
    b. 5
    c. 6
    d. 7

263. If a prescription contains any filthy substance or could have been contaminated, then it is considered

     a. Adultered
     b. Misbranded
     c. Both A and B

264. Which of the following is not required on a Schedule II prescription

     a. Quantity – written as a number and a word
     b. Patient's age or date of birth
     c. Intended use
     d. All are required

265. Which classes of pharmacy must be represented by pharmacist members of the board

     a. Class A
     b. Class B
     c. Class C
     d. All of the above
     e. A and C only

266. The process of affixing a label, including all information required by federal and state statute or regulation, to a drug or device container is referred to as

     a. Label
     b. Labeling
     c. Unit dose packaging

267. Drug samples for dangerous drugs are allowed to be dispensed from a Class D pharmacy

a. True
b. False

268. A clinic pharmacy is considered which class of pharmacy

   a. Class D
   b. Class E
   c. Class F
   d. Class G
   e. Class H

Answers

1. A	22. B	43. C
2. D	23. A	44. C
3. C	24. A	45. B
4. B	25. C	46. B
5. B	26. B	47. A
6. E	27. C	48. E
7. C	28. C	49. C
8. A	29. A	50. D
9. E	30. C	51. D
10. C	31. B	52. C
11. D	32. C	53. B
12. D	33. E	54. A
13. B	34. C	55. D
14. B	35. A	56. C
15. B	36. A	57. B
16. B	37. A	58. C
17. D	38. D	59. A
18. A	39. E	60. B
19. B	40. A	61. A
20. C	41. E	62. D
21. B	42. B	63. C

64. D	88. C	112. B
65. B	89. D	113. B
66. H	90. A	114. C
67. B	91. A	115. E
68. C	92. B	116. A
69. C	93. B	117. C
70. C	94. C	118. B
71. C	95. C	119. B
72. A	96. D	120. C
73. D	97. C	121. B
74. E	98. B	122. B
75. C	99. A	123. D
76. A	100. C	124. A
77. B	101. C	125. A
78. B	102. C	126. A
79. A	103. B	127. B
80. A	104. B	128. A
81. C	105. B	129. B
82. D	106. C	130. D
83. D	107. C	131. D
84. A	108. B	132. A
85. A	109. D	133. A
86. B	110. B	134. A
87. A	111. B	135. A

136. E	160. D	184. B
137. D	161. D	185. C
138. D	162. D	186. A
139. B	163. A	187. A
140. C	164. D	188. E
141. A	165. D	189. B
142. D	166. A	190. C
143. A	167. A	191. B
144. D	168. A	192. A
145. B	169. E	193. C
146. B	170. D	194. B
147. A	171. B	195. C
148. D	172. B	196. A
149. C	173. D	197. D
150. B	174. D	198. B
151. B	175. B	199. C
152. A	176. B	200. A
153. D	177. B	201. D
154. B	178. A	202. A
155. D	179. A	203. A
156. B	180. C	204. B
157. C	181. D	205. B
158. C	182. B	206. B
159. D	183. B	207. A

208. B	229. D	250. D
209. D	230. B	251. B
210. B	231. D	252. C
211. D	232. A	253. A
212. C	233. D	254. B
213. B	234. C	255. B
214. B	235. A	256. C
215. D	236. D	257. D
216. D	237. D	258. C
217. B	238. A	259. D
218. A	239. A	260. A
219. E	240. B	261. C
220. B	241. B	262. D
221. A	242. C	263. A
222. C	243. B	264. D
223. D	244. A	265. E
224. B	245. D	266. B
225. D	246. D	267. A
226. B	247. B	268. A
227. A	248. D	
228. C	249. D	

Made in the USA
Lexington, KY
27 March 2015